Rhinosinusitis

Edited by Balwant Singh Gendeh and Mirjana Turkalj

Published in London, United Kingdom

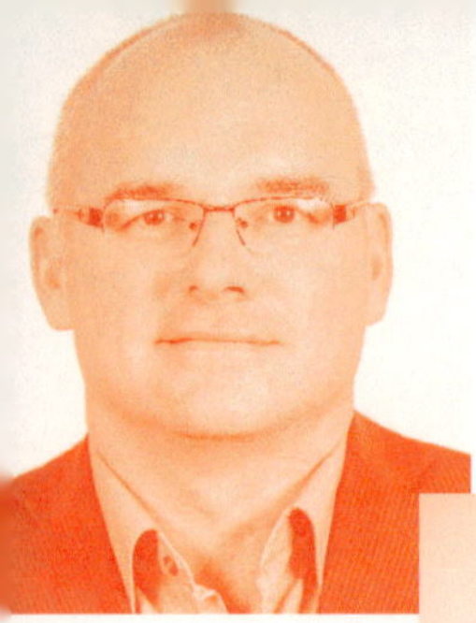
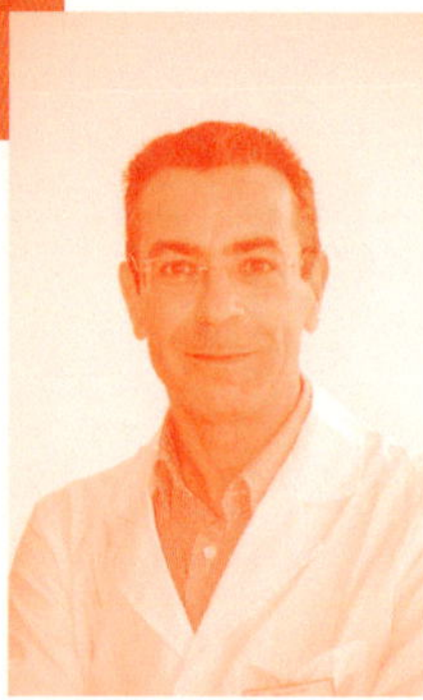
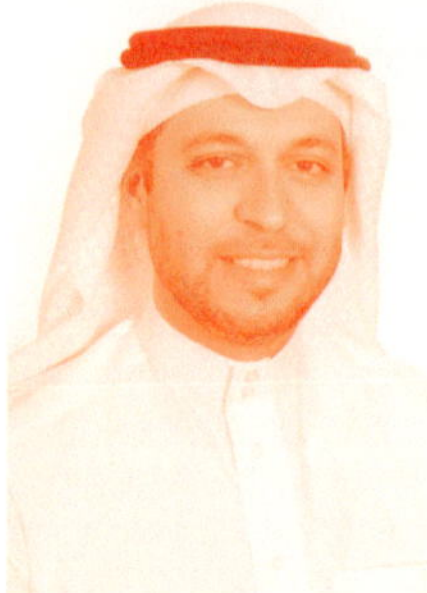
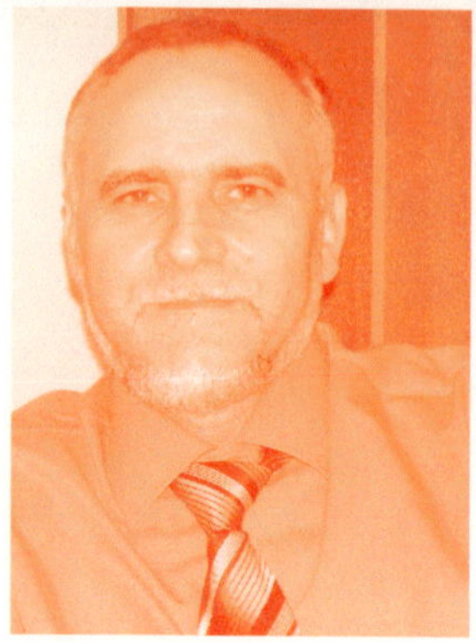
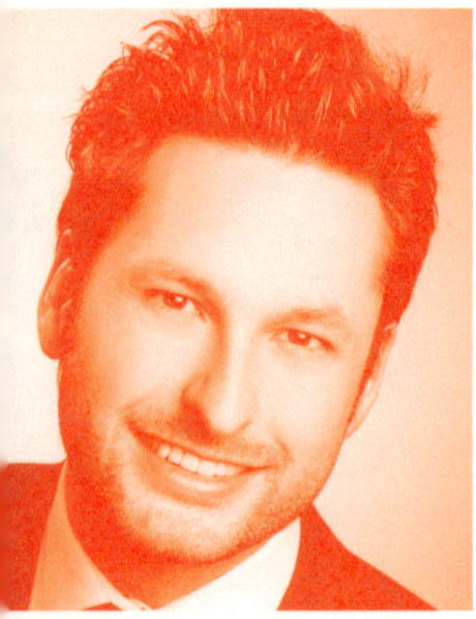
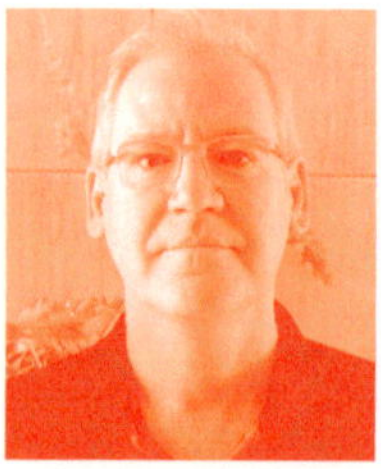
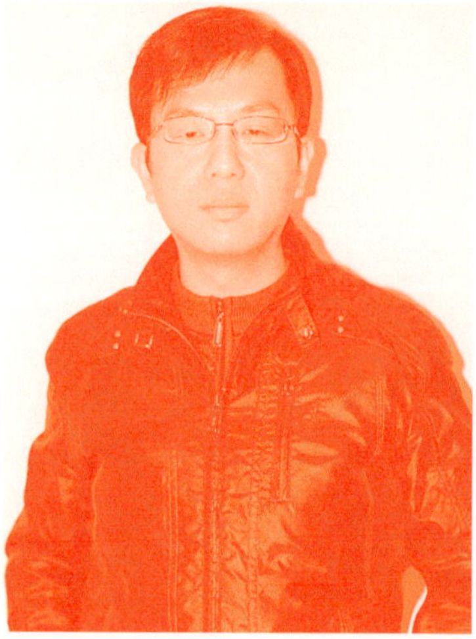

IntechOpen

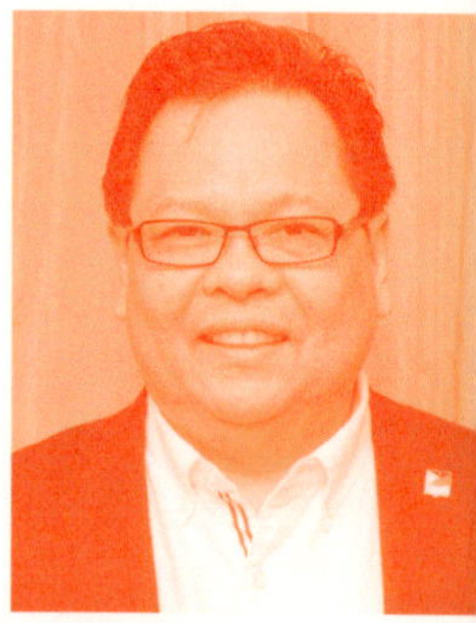
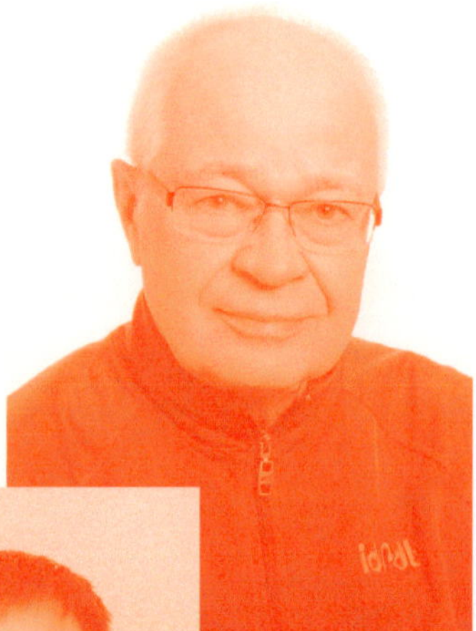
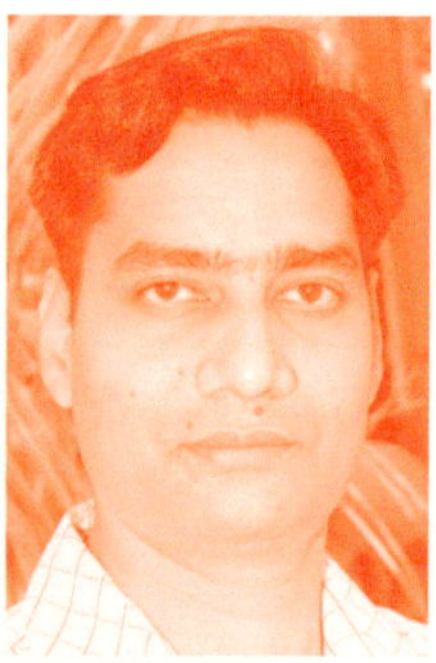
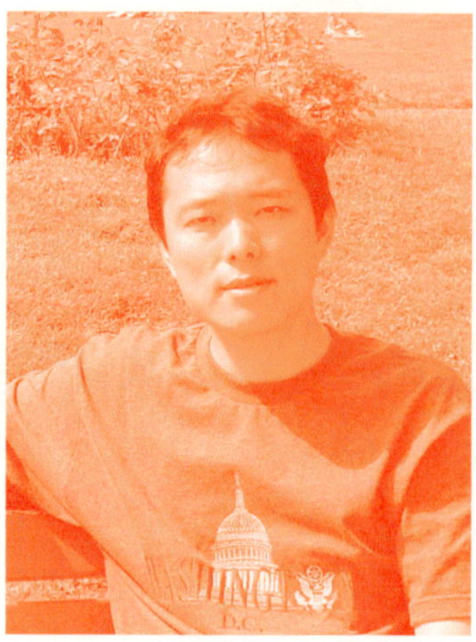
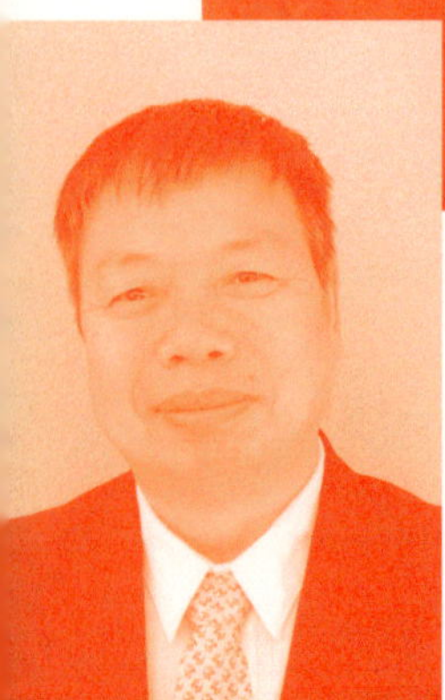
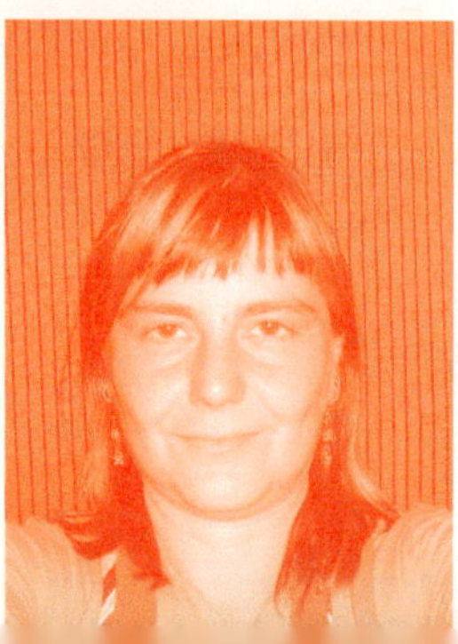

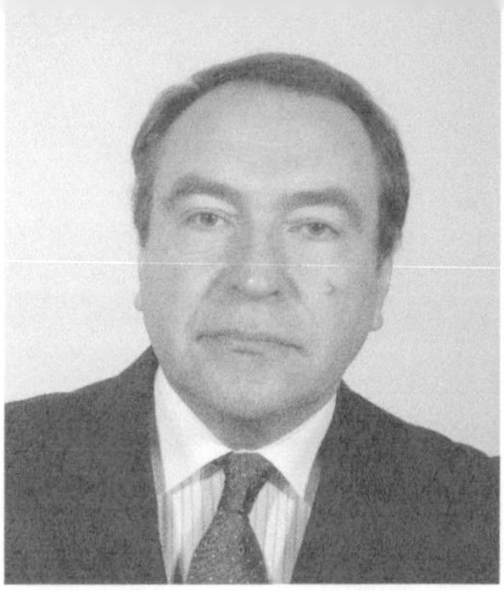

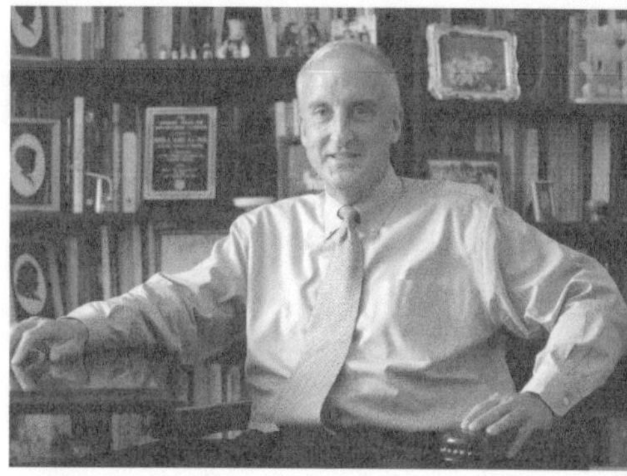

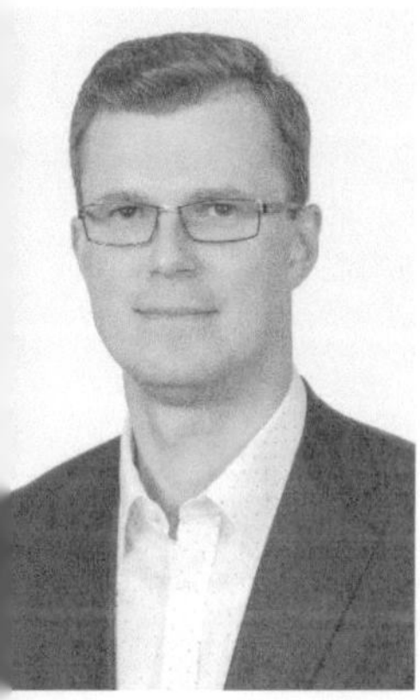

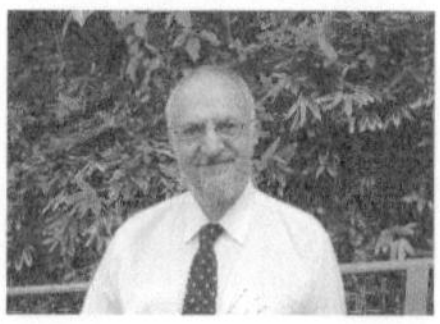

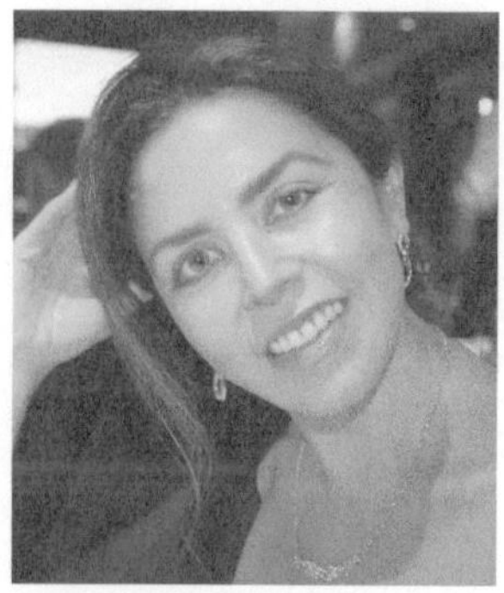

Supporting open minds since 2005

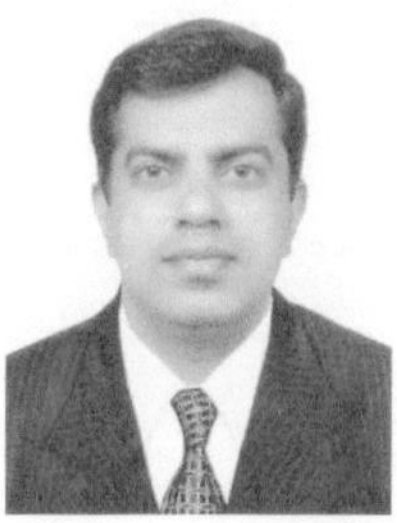

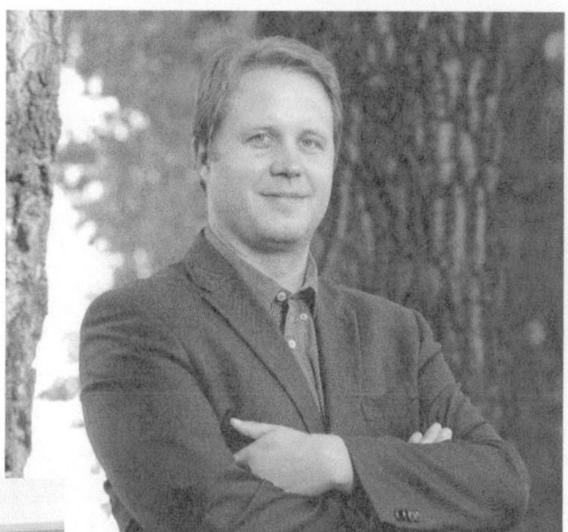

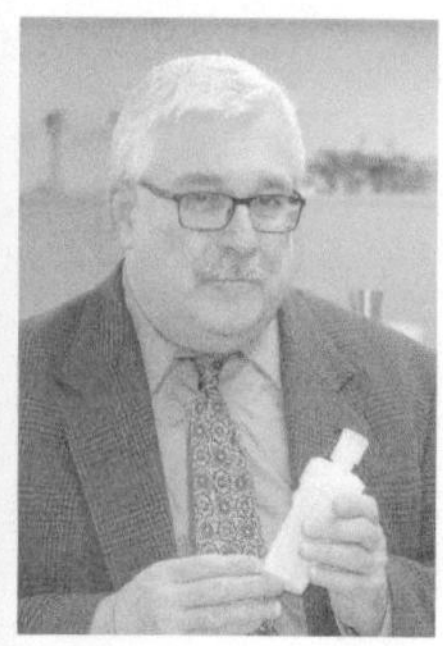

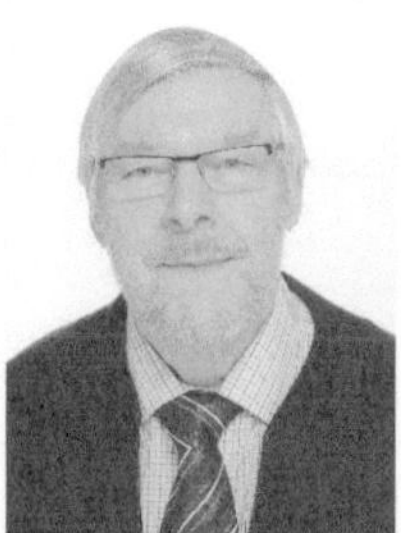

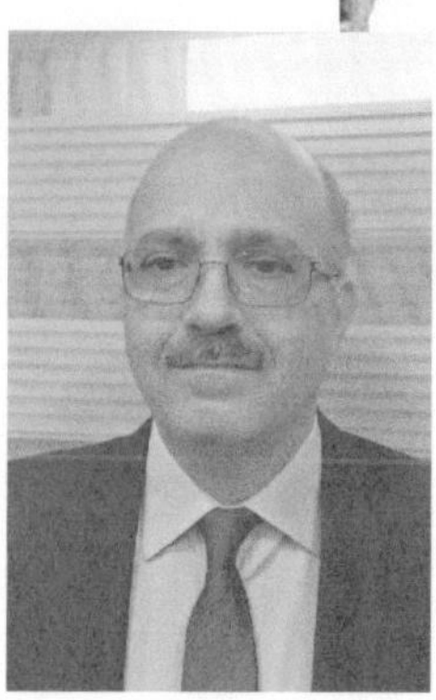

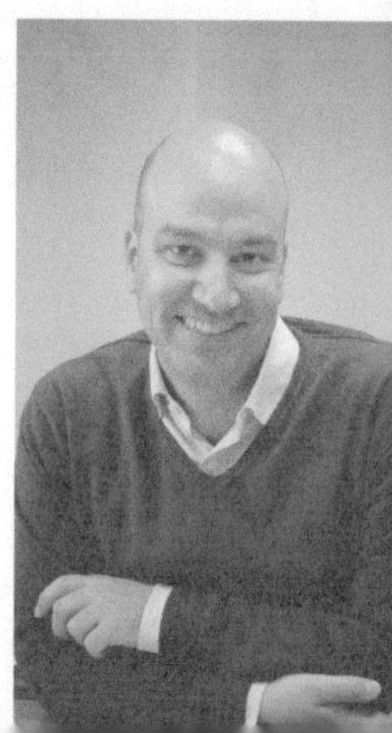

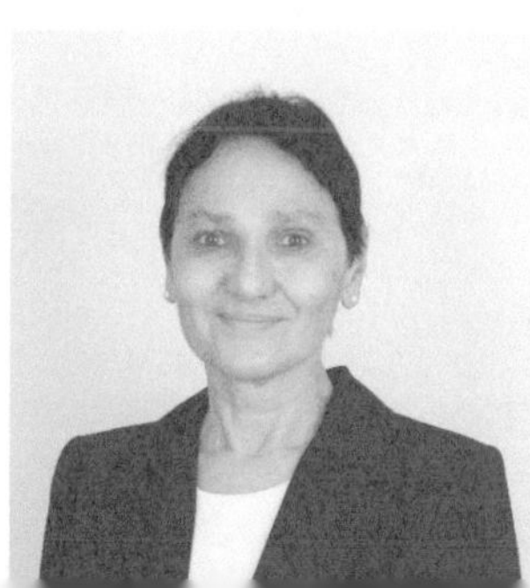

Rhinosinusitis
http://dx.doi.org/10.5772/intechopen.73825
Edited by Balwant Singh Gendeh and Mirjana Turkalj

Contributors
Zeinab AlQudehy, Lena Telmsani, Te-Huei Yeh, Yi-Tsen Lin, Balwant Singh Gendeh, Giampiero Neri, Fiorella Cazzato, Pasquina La Torre, Lucia Centurione, Elisa Vestrini, Giampaolo Quaternato, Letizia Neri, Gennady Fedorovitch, Marco Capelli, Bogdan Nowicki, Alexander Nowicki, Natalie Nowicki, Stella Nowicki, Alfred Samet, Roger Su, James K. Fortson, Michał Michalik, Shrikant Phatak, Richa Agrawal, Blaženka Kljaić Bukvić, Mario Blekić, Marija Pečnjak, Ramit Maoz-Segal, Diti Machnes-Maayan, Irena Veksler-Offengenden, Soad Hajyahia, Shirly Frizinsky, Nancy Agmon-Levin, Andrew Kiboneka, Dan Kibuule

First published in London, United Kingdom, 2019 by IntechOpen
IntechOpen is the global imprint of INTECHOPEN LIMITED, registered in England and Wales, registration number: 11086078, 7th floor, 10 Lower Thames Street, London, EC3R 6AF, United Kingdom
Printed in Croatia

British Library Cataloguing-in-Publication Data
A catalogue record for this book is available from the British Library

Additional hard and PDF copies can be obtained from orders@intechopen.com

Rhinosinusitis
Edited by Balwant Singh Gendeh and Mirjana Turkalj
p. cm.
Print ISBN 978-1-78984-043-8
Online ISBN 978-1-78984-044-5
eBook (PDF) ISBN 978-1-83968-007-6

For EU product safety concerns:
IN TECH d.o.o., Prolaz Marije Krucifikse Kozulić 3, 51000 Rijeka, Croatia, info@intechopen.com or visit our website at intechopen.com.

Meet the editors

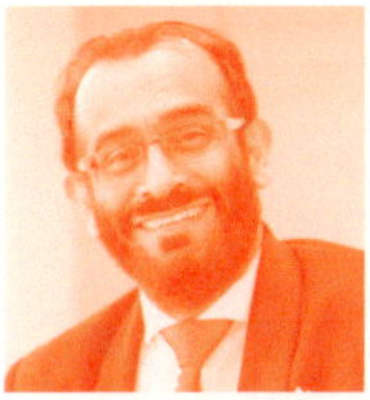

Dr. Balwant Singh Gendeh is a senior consultant ENT surgeon with subspecialty interest in rhinology (allergies, sinonasal diseases, endoscopic sinus, anterior and ventral skull base surgery, and functional and cosmetic nasal surgery). He was an ENT registrar at the Royal Infirmary, Middlesbrough, UK, in 1993 and subsequently a JW Fulbright scholar at the University of Pittsburgh, USA, in 1997. During his Fulbright experience, he also worked at the Hospital of the University of Pennsylvania, Philadelphia, and St. Joseph's Hospital, Chicago, USA, with subspecialty interest in rhinology and aesthetic nasal surgery. Dr. Gendeh retired as a consultant ENT surgeon at the National University of Malaysia Medical Centre (UKMMC) in 2014, and presently is a visiting professor at the Department of Otorhinolaryngology-Head and Neck Surgery at UKMMC. He has also been a resident ENT consultant at Pantai Hospital Kuala Lumpur since 2014. Due to his vast contribution to academia in research and clinical publications, he was elected as a Diploma of the Fellowship Academy of Medicine Malaysia in October 2000, International Fellow of the Academy of Otolaryngology Head and Neck Surgery in April 2004, Fellow of the Academy of Sciences Malaysia in April 2016, and Fellow of the Malaysian Scientific Association in September 2017.

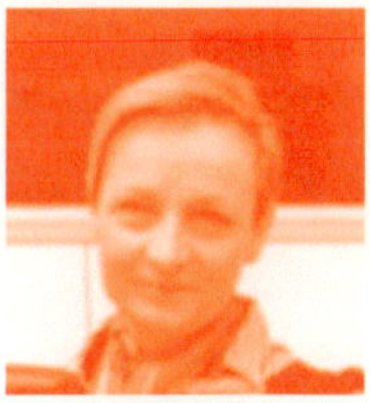

Assoc. Prof. Mirjana Turkalj, MD, PhD, graduated from the Faculty of Medicine in Zagreb. Since 1998 she has been a pediatric specialist, and from 2005 a subspecialist in allergology and clinical immunology, and pulmonology. She was elected scientific assistant professor in 2015, and acquired the title of associate professor in 2017. She works as a pediatric subspecialist at Srebrnjak Children's Hospital in Zagreb, where she is also Deputy Director, Head of the Clinical Allergology Center of the Croatian Ministry of Health, and Head of the Department for Allergology, Immunology, and Pulmonology. Mirjana is a lecturer at the Faculty of Medicine, University of Zagreb, and University of Osijek, Faculty of Food Technology and Biotechnology, Faculty of Pharmacy and Biochemistry, and Catholic University of Croatia. She is a member of the European Academy of Allergology and Clinical Immunology, the European Respiratory Society, the Croatian Medical Association, the Croatian Society for Pediatric Pathology, the Croatian Society for Health Ecology, and many others. Her medical interests are immunological mechanisms in asthma and allergic diseases, pathomechanisms of allergen-specific immunotherapy, the role of infections in the development of allergies, and prevention of allergic diseases in children. She has written more than 190 scientific papers with more than 400 citations, and 16 book chapters.

Contents

Preface

This book covers selected topics on rhinosinusitis, which provides a journey into advancements in various aspects of the field. A collection of manuscripts of this nature involves extensive exposure and accumulation of knowledge from experience collected over many years and covers both basic and clinical concepts of upper and lower airway problems affecting health. Each author has contributed his/her own perspective on each topic, adding theories, future trends, and research findings.

The chapters of this book are arranged under five sections, namely Allergic Rhinitis, Sinusitis, Dental Related Sinusitis, One Airway Disease, and Surgical Techniques in Sino-Nasal Diseases. This book is intended for general otolaryngologists, rhinologists, immunologists, allergologists, pulmonologists in subspecialty-related fields, researchers, and fellows to arouse innovative new ideas for future basic research in clinical practice.

This publication is the outcome of input from multinational-related, one airway-related specialties from all over the globe with the common goal of better human health care. Some of the authors are very experienced, while others are newcomers such as researches or clinicians.

This book is accessible online to allow free access to as many readers as possible and is available in print for those who do not have internet access or are interested in having their own hard copy. Hopefully, this publication will contribute to the global distribution of knowledge in one airway disease affecting the nose, sinuses, and lungs.

We would like to congratulate each and every one of the contributors for his/her excellent input on each chapter and the valuable time and effort taken in contributing to the completion of this book.

We would like to thank Ms. Sandra Maljavac, the Author Service Manager, for her expert assistance on all issues concerning the book; Ms. Sandra Bakic, the Commissioning Editor, for her tireless assistance; and all those for choosing me to be the editor and Associate Professor Dr. Mirjana Turkalj as co-editor of this book. My kind gratitude goes to the technical editors for arranging the book in a uniform format and IntechOpen for undertaking this novel mission.

We would like to thank our valuable teachers from whom we have gained knowledge throughout the years. Lastly, but not least, we would like to dedicate this book to our spouses, children, and loved ones for all their patience and understanding.

We hope that this book will be part of a series of books in all subspecialties involving one airway disease and that it will enhance global collaboration not only between physicians but also for the betterment of humankind. We wish readers an enjoyable journey and hope they find this book interesting.

Balwant Singh Gendeh MBBS (Kashmir), MS (ORL-HNS) UKM, AM (Mal), FAMM, FASc (M'sia), FMSA
Visiting Professor and Senior Consultant ENT Surgeon/Rhinologist (Endoscopic Sinus/Skull Base Surgery and Functional and Cosmetic Nasal Surgery), Department of Otorhinolaryngology-Head Neck Surgery (ORL-HNS), UKMMC and Resident ENT Surgeon, Pantai Hospital Kuala Lumpur, Malaysia

Mirjana Turkalj MD, MSc, PhD
Associate Professor,
Deputy Director,
Department of Pulmonology,
Allergology and Immunology,
Srebrnjak Children's Hospital,
Zagreb, Croatia

Section 1

Allergic Rhinitis

Chapter 1

Allergic March

Blaženka Kljaić Bukvić, Mario Blekić and Marija Pečnjak

Abstract

Atopy is an inherited tendency of producing immunoglobulin E on common proteins from the environment like pollen, house mites and food. The presence of atopy represents a risk for the development of allergic diseases like atopic dermatitis, asthma, allergic rhinitis and food allergy, although atopy can also be present only in the form of asymptomatic sensitization. Allergic diseases share common inherited and environmental risk factors, immunologic patterns of allergen-specific Th2 response and efferent phase of immunologic reaction characterized with the production of IgE and activation of granulocytes. The presence of one disease increases the risk for developing other diseases. Allergic diseases demonstrate characteristic sequence of incidence in childhood which is called allergic/atopic march and starts with atopic dermatitis in early infancy. Disrupted integrity of the skin in atopic dermatitis contributes to the development of sensitization and increases the risk for development of other allergic diseases. The discovery of filaggrin gene mutation opens the possibility for causative incidence of allergic diseases and for prevention of development of atopic march. But, the causal link from atopic dermatitis to asthma is still a matter of debate.

Keywords: allergic march, atopy, children

1. Introduction

Allergic diseases are the most common chronic condition in childhood. Epidemiological studies observed increase in the prevalence of allergic diseases from the middle of the twentieth century, which is explained by environment and lifestyle changes and improvements in modern Westernized societies. At the beginning of the twenty-first century, stagnation in the prevalence of asthma while increase in the prevalence of food allergy was noticed, which announced the second wave of allergy epidemics [1–3]. The first atopic phenotype that starts in early infancy is atopic dermatitis (AD). It is estimated that it affects up to 20% of children. Disrupted integrity of the skin barrier contributes to the development of sensitization to food and aeroallergens and also increases the risk for the development of food allergy. It is considered that 30% of children with AD have food allergy, and 30% develop asthma and 75% allergic rhinitis [4]. About 3–5% of children have been diagnosed with food allergy, and up to 50% of them have AD [1]. AD and food allergy can coexist and can also appear independently in infancy and in the first years of life. In the following years, wheezing induced by viruses like respiratory syncytial virus or rhinovirus and sensitization to inhalational allergens can be observed. As the child grows up, respiratory symptoms are more common and occur outside of the infection; introduction of anti-inflammatory drugs is needed, i.e., the signs of asthma occur. Preschool and school age are the time of appearance of allergic sensitization to pollen of grass, weed and tree pollen, and the beginning of allergic rhinoconjunctivitis which persists in adolescence and the young adult age.

At the same time, remission of atopic dermatitis and food allergy is noticed, while asthma and rhinitis symptoms continue. Sensitizations to pollen and cross-reactions to nuts, fresh fruits and vegetables may induce oral allergy syndrome, the type of food allergy that occurs in the school age. Asthma may disappear in teenage years, but after some period of remission, skin and respiratory symptoms can appear once again. In early adulthood, skin and lung symptoms are related to tobacco smoking, occupational exposures and lifestyle, and they manifest like contact dermatitis or asthma-chronic obstructive pulmonary disease overlap syndrome [5].

Atopic dermatitis, food allergy, asthma and allergic rhinitis in childhood share the common genetic, epigenetic and environmental risk factors, while the underpinning pathogenesis is marked with disrupted skin, lung and gut barriers, altered microbiome and local and systemic Th-2-driven immunological pathways. Those allergic conditions can comanifest or occur in temporal sequence. The hypothesis that has been proposed to clarify time sequence and associations of allergic disease is called allergic march. This concept means that allergic disorder starts in early infancy with the first hallmark of atopy and atopic dermatitis and then appears food allergy, and later in childhood comes asthma and allergic rhinitis. Some investigators presumed that the underlying allergic inflammation of the skin could progress from atopic dermatitis to asthma. In addition, some preventive measures like improving skin barrier before skin disease onset can reduce the risk for respiratory allergy. Those observations support the causal link between atopic dermatitis and asthma. Although described longitudinal appearance of all allergic diseases was noticed only in small proportion (~7%) of children [6, 7], others had different trajectories of one or more allergic diseases which can occur in different point of time in childhood. Last explanations are talking about a cluster of coexistence-related allergic diseases rather than a progression.

2. Atopic dermatitis, disrupted skin barrier and allergic sensitization: is it the beginning?

Atopic dermatitis is the most common chronic skin disorder in childhood. It appears in early childhood with dry, itchy skin and eczema on the cheeks, wrists and other parts of the body. Up to 20% of children experience AD in childhood. The majority outgrows eczema, but one proportion of them continues to have symptoms into adulthood [8]. According to the recently published cohort, six latent classes representing subphenotypes of AD were identified. These classes can be summarized in four classes as follows: unaffected individual or transient AD (61.9%); early-onset-persistent AD (10.7%); early-onset late resolving, early-onset early resolving and mid-onset resolving by age 11 years of age (16.5%); and later-onset AD after age 3.5 years (10.9%) [9].

AD is a systemic disorder characterized by disrupted skin barrier. It is considered that factors associated with damage of skin barrier are complex and influenced by a combination of structural, genetic, environmental and immunological factors. Structural changes are caused by altered lipid composition, decreased structural proteins, increased skin pH and reduced skin microbiome diversity. Cutaneous permeability defects can be assessed by measuring transepidermal water loss (TEWL) which correlates with disease severity. Several genetic defects encoding skin barrier proteins contribute to the breakdown of skin barrier. Inherited loss-of-function mutations in filaggrin gene, which encodes structural epidermis proteins, are associated with early-onset AD that is more often persistent and closely related with asthma and food allergy [10]. Polymorphisms in the thymic stromal lymphopoietin (TSLP) gene, SPINK5 gene and corneodesmosin have also been linked to AD and the development of food allergy [11–13]. The inflammatory responses induced by AD are manifested by increased production of Th2 cytokines such as IL-4, IL-13, IL-25, IL-33 and TSLP. TSLP is one of the major inductors of systemic Th2 response, and it is considered that it could be the link between skin and respiratory allergy. It is expressed in skin keratinocytes, pulmonary airway and intestinal epithelium, while increased expression was observed in the skin of AD patients and respiratory epithelium of asthma patients [14].

Skin microbiome dysbiosis is characterized by the dominance of *Staphylococcus aureus* which through various mechanisms worsens chronic skin inflammation [15]. Skin barrier dysfunction is associated with innate immune activation that results in dysregulated immune response to environmental antigens (like allergens and bacteria) and skin inflammation leading to the evolution of allergic sensitization [16]. Several studies on animals and humans support the concept that damaged skin promotes sensitizations. In mouse, exposure to egg and peanuts through disrupted skin induces sensitization [17] and, after exposure to egg aerosol, could induce asthma-like airway hyperresponsiveness [18]. In children, applications of peanut oil to inflamed skin were positively associated with the development of peanut food allergies [19], and the use of wheat-containing facial soap was positively associated with the development of wheat food allergy [20]. Application of oat-based creams on the skin of children with AD can induce oat sensitization in one third of children [21]. The concept of allergic march has been supported by cross-sectional and longitudinal birth cohort studies. Several birth cohorts have shown associations between early-onset AD and development of asthma and allergic rhinitis in school age [22, 23]; risk is greater in children with early-onset persistent AD phenotype [24]. Children with AD and allergic sensitization had increased risk of food allergy, asthma and allergic rhinitis compared to non-sensitized children without AD [25]. Food sensitizations in the first 2 years of life were associated with increased risk of asthma and allergic rhinitis in school age [26]. Peanut, milk and egg food allergy also increased the risk of developing asthma and rhinitis later in childhood [27]. Meta-analyses of birth cohort studies which investigated atopic march observed that early-life food sensitization was associated with an increased risk of infantile eczema, childhood wheeze/asthma, eczema and allergic rhinitis and young adult asthma [28].

The development of sensitization is complex, and except skin barrier defect and environmental allergen exposure, the presence of other factors is important because they may function as adjuvants, and some of them are bacterial colonization of the skin, allergens with intrinsic protease activity and exogenous adjuvants [29].

3. Why is allergy increasing? Hypothesis-driven strategy

Allergic diseases of the skin, gut and lung are complex disorders with multiple phenotypes and underlying genotypes. They occur as a result of environmental exposures during early life in individuals with genetic susceptibility to allergy. Gene-environment interactions are accountable for different influences of the environment on individual level. There are several hypotheses of allergy increase in the twentieth century. According to the *hygiene hypothesis*, decreased exposure to microorganisms in modern society, through increased hygiene and decreased prevalence of infection in early life, disrupts immune tolerance and directs immunological reaction toward Th2 direction [30].

The beginning of hygiene hypothesis can be found in the David Strachan study from 1989. He observed that children who grew up in large families, with large number of older siblings, have less allergy and concluded that exposure to infection in early life (prenatally and early childhood) can prevent allergy [31]. This was confirmed by subsequent studies which linked less allergies with viral, bacterial or protozoic pathogens, transmitted by the fecal-oral route [32]. In 1990 hygiene hypothesis was supported by the observation that growing up on farms, regular contact with farm animals, stables and drinking unpasteurized milk were protective against allergy [33]. Farms are microbe-rich environment. Endotoxin, lipopolysaccharide, part of the outer layer of Gram-negative bacteria, is a marker of microbe surroundings. Its protective effect on atopy is produced by stimulation of immune system in Th1 direction. Preventive effect of endotoxin was seen only for early-life exposure (prenatal and early childhood, before development of allergic sensitization) [33, 34].

In the past 20 years, hygiene hypothesis was expanded by "old friends hypothesis" and "biodiversity hypothesis" [35, 36]. According to that hypothesis, contact with natural environment and its species (included microbes and parasites) protects against allergy. Children are exposed to the environment indirectly (through mother during prenatal life) and directly through the skin, gut and lung. Changes in the microbiome of the gut, skin and nose reduced microbiome diversity, and loss of symbiotic relationship with parasites and bacteria increased the risk for allergic disease [37]. Stability and diversity of gut microbiome are developed during early life (first 1000 days of postnatal life). This process can be influenced with different factors like mode of birth, infant feeding, fiber content in the mother's and child's diet and older siblings and exposure to pets and/or farm animals during childhood. Environment and dietary habits of mother and previous generations can change microbe diversity of neonate's trough epigenetic modification [38–42].

The second hypothesis *dual-allergen exposure hypothesis* is based on observations that allergic sensitization occurs through disrupted skin in AD, while early ingestion of food (before development of sensitization) allows development of oral tolerance [43]. Delayed introduction of solid food in infancy, which were recommended at the end of the twentieth was not protective for food allergy development [44]. This hypothesis was confirmed by several randomized clinical trials like Learning Early About Peanut Allergy (LEAP) and Enquiring About Tolerance (EAT). EAT was looking at the early introduction of six common food allergens at 3 months of age alongside breastfeeding compared to exclusive breastfed infants. It found that prevalence of egg allergy was lower among infants with early introduction [45]. LEAP assessed oral tolerance induction of peanut in group of high-risk infants between 4 and 11 months of age. It compared early and regular peanut consumption, average of 6 grams of peanut protein a week, in relation to completely avoiding peanut protein until 60 months of age. Early introduction of peanut protein results in significant reduction in peanut allergy. LEAP-On study was an extension of LEAP, in which protective effect of early introduction on peanut allergy was observed, even after cessation of peanut consumption [46, 47]. According to the findings from the studies like LEAP and EAT, guidelines for complementary feeding were remarkably changed. Pediatric and allergy societies have published consensus statements about early introduction of peanuts in high-risk infants. Also, current recommendations advise against delayed introduction of allergenic food into infant diet [48, 49].

Recent researches report about the important role of vitamin D in the pathogenesis of allergy. Vitamin D has positive impact on foetal lung development and an immunomodulatory effect; it stimulates differentiation of T lymphocytes, induction of Treg, while its deficiency induces Th2 response [50]. It was observed that rise in allergy prevalence occurs with increasing *vitamin D deficiency* especially among populations less exposed to the sun [51]. Deficit of vitamin D is associated with increased risk of peanut and egg food allergy, atopic dermatitis and asthma. The severe form of the diseases was observed with higher vitamin D deficiency [52, 53].

4. Allergic march: causal link or cluster of related diseases

The allergic march is a real phenomenon, but there is a great debate about underlying mechanisms. Some researchers argue that there is a causal link between AD and other allergic diseases in childhood, in which AD is the first disease with local and systemic immunological response. Systemic response could trigger multisystem allergic disease. Longitudinal, prospective population-based cohorts or cohorts of high-risk infants reported about increased risk of asthma and allergic rhinitis among children with previous or current AD [54–59].

Meta-analysis of 13 prospective birth cohort studies reported that odd ratio of asthma among children with AD in the first 4 years of life was 2.14% (95% CI 1.67–2.75), while the prevalence of asthma at the age of 6 years in eczema cohort studies was 29.5% (95% CI, 28.2–32.7%). The conclusion was that only one in every three children with eczema develops asthma during later childhood [4]. According to the results of high-risk birth cohort, 26.7% children with AD developed AR at 7 years of age, while the risk is higher among children with persistent and late-onset AD (OR 2.68, 95% CI 0.97–7.41) [57]. Sensitization to food allergen increased the risk for AR (OR 1.2, 95% CI 0.6–2.2), but the associations is stronger among children who had co-sensitization to both food and aeroallergens (OR 3.1, 95% CI 1.2–7.8) [28]. In the PASTURE study, children with early-persistent AD phenotype and those with late phenotype had an increased risk of developing allergic rhinitis. Early AD phenotype did not associate with AR, while the risk increased among children with early AD and food allergy [60]. According to these results, there was a new question: can we predict which phenotype of AD will be linked to asthma? More information come from longitudinal cohorts which analyzed different phenotypes of AD based on disease course and determined which classes are at highest risk for other atopic diseases [9, 60, 61]. According to the results from those studies, the early-onset, severe, persistent phenotype is associated with the highest risk for allergic comorbidities. Polysensitization, atopic heredity and filaggrin loss-of-mutation contribute to increased risk [62]. Children with high-risk phenotype of AD are candidates for preventive measures, which could delay or stop the occurrence of asthma and allergic rhinitis. But, it is considered that there is not enough evidence that AD causes asthma and allergic rhinitis. Paller et al., in recent review, presumed existence of inherited predisposition to one or more atopic disorders. Occurrence of the disease is a result of complex interplay between different underlying genotypes and environmental exposures during maturation of immune system, with tissue-specific peak time of clinical manifestation. Allergic diseases have different phenotypes and different trajectories that form clusters [62].

Simultaneously with AR, local allergic rhinitis (LAR) can appear in the preschool age. This entity of rhinitis is marked with local synthesis of specific IgE but without systemic allergy (allergic sensitizations and specific IgE). It was observed that LAR is a separate, well-defined phenotype of noninfectious rhinitis, which is stable over time [63, 64]. But, among younger patients and children, LAR can be the first step in the natural evolution to classical AR, especially when starting in the first two decades of life and in polysensitized patients [65]. In the German Multicentric Allergy Study, it was observed that over one third of the children developing a typical grass pollen-related seasonal AR had no serum-specific IgE to pollen. These children develop a systemic IgE sensitization to grass pollens in the second or third pollen season following the onset of their rhinitis symptoms [66, 67]. If patients with LAR have AR over time, this supports atopic march.

5. Can we prevent and/or stop atopic march?

Better understanding of underpinning mechanisms of atopic dermatitis and atopic comorbidities as well as environmental risk factors induces further researches of preventive interventions aimed at stopping atopic march. Those interventions could be started during pregnancy and early life among healthy or high-risk infants before onset of disease (primary prevention) or among children with one atopic disease in order to prevent appearance of other atopic comorbidities (secondary prevention).

Disrupted skin barriers promote sensitizations and increase the risk for allergic disease. Improvement in skin barrier through regular application of emollients beginning in the neonatal period can prevent AD among high-risk children. Protective effect was observed if treatment lasted up to 6–8 months of age [68–70]. There was favorable effect at the 12 months of age, even after treatment was ceased [69]. These researches support original hypothesis of skin barrier dysfunction as a beginning of atopy march, but it is still unclear if this protective effect is long-lasting or onset of AD is delayed. The effect of emollients on food allergy was unclear. Only one research showed a trend for decreased food sensitization at 6 and 12 months of age [69], while two other were not powered to measure food sensitization [68, 70]. Some of undergoing studies aim to investigate the effect of emollients in prevention of AD among general population.

Local and system inflammatory response is a hallmark of AD, and anti-inflammatory therapy is effective in control of exacerbations, but study of Schneider et al. showed ineffectiveness of pimecrolimus in stopping atopic march [71]. Skin microbiome dysbiosis can increase the risk for onset or exacerbation of AD and comorbidities [72]. Recent researches showed that topical application of skin commensal bacteria can improve lesions in AD [73, 74]. Apart from local use of bacteria, the great interest of researchers is the role of probiotics in protection of allergy. Several studies have shown positive effect of probiotics like that adding *Lactobacillus rhamnosus* in diet of pregnant women can reduce the risk of AD [75]. Adding probiotics like *Bifidobacterium lactis*, *Lactobacillus salivarius* or *Lactobacillus GG* to the infant formula reduced the severity of AD [76]. But recent randomized control trial has shown opposite result. The study concluded that early supplementation with LGG in the first 6 months of life does not appear to prevent eczema at 2 years of age [77]. However, systematic reviews and meta-analyses report protective effect of the probiotics for the primary prevention of atopic dermatitis [78–80]. Probiotics are ineffective in prevention of asthma, food allergy and allergic rhinitis. Medical societies like the American Academy of Pediatrics, the European Academy of Allergy and Clinical Immunology and the European Society for Pediatric Gastroenterology, Hepatology and Nutrition do not recommend the use of probiotics for primary prevention of allergic disease [49, 81–83]. The World Allergy Organization recommends the use of probiotics in diet of mothers of high-risk infants during pregnancy and lactation and in diet of those infants in order to prevent AD [84]. There is no consensus for the most effective specific strain of probiotics. The strain, dosage, timing of introduction and duration of probiotics usage are still uncertain. These questions are the aim of the future investigations.

Early introduction of allergenic food like peanut and egg can prevent food allergy, but the effect on other allergic diseases is not known. Exposure to furry pets in home like dogs and cats in early life can prevent sensitization, but this protective effect can be modified by endotoxin exposure [85]. Deficiency of vitamin D has been associated with onset and exacerbation of allergy. According to this immunomodulatory effect, it has been assumed that supplementation of vitamin D might protect against allergy. But recent researches does not support protective role of vitamin D in allergy [86, 87].

In the prevention of allergic diseases, protective effect was observed for antihistamines. In infants with atopic dermatitis or with high risk for allergy, ketotifen treatment was associated with lower incidence of asthma [88], while the use of cetirizine decreased the risk for asthma in grass pollen-sensitized children [89]. Allergen immunotherapy (AIT) has been used over the last 100 years and is the only therapy with disease-modifying effect. The role of AIT in primary and secondary prevention was investigated in several studies. Sublingual AIT applied for the primary prevention of allergy among high-risk infants has no protective effect on the developing of first allergic disease [90]. Oral AIT decreased the risk of asthma, among children with grass pollen allergic rhinitis [91]. Recent systematic review and meta-analysis found no evidence that AIT decreased the risk for developing a first allergic disease. However, AIT reduced the risk of asthma among patients with allergic rhinitis. This effect was observed 2 and more years after the AIT was completed. AIT can reduce the onset of new sensitizations, but the evidence was not clear [92, 93].

6. Conclusion

Allergic diseases like atopic dermatitis, asthma and allergic rhinitis have sequential appearance with typical peaks of incidence during childhood. This temporal association is observed in the whole children population, and it starts with atopic dermatitis and food allergy in infancy, followed with asthma in the preschool age and finishes with allergic rhinitis. During growing up, the remission of atopic dermatitis and asthma was noticed, while symptoms of allergic rhinitis persist through adolescence and young adult age. The occurrence of all allergy diseases among the same child in temporal appearance was noticed only in smaller proportion of children in which causal link between AD, asthma and AR can be presumed; while, among others, common occurrence of allergic diseases follows different trajectories, without typical allergic sequence. For those children, complex interplay of allergic predisposition, systemic and local immunological responses and environmental influences during maturation of immune system triggers the appearance of those coexistence of allergic disease.

Author details

Blaženka Kljaić Bukvić[1,2,3*], Mario Blekić[1,2,3] and Marija Pečnjak[1]

1 Pediatric Department, General Hospital "Dr. Josip Benčević", Croatia

2 School of Medicine, Josip Juraj Strossmayer University of Osijek, Osijek, Croatia

3 Faculty of Dental Medicine and Health Care, Josip Juraj Strossmayer University of Osijek, Osijek, Croatia

*Address all correspondence to: blazenka.bukvic@gmail.com

References

[1] Boyce JA et al. Guidelines for the diagnosis and management of food allergy in the United States: Summary of the NIAID-sponsored expert panel report. The Journal of Allergy and Clinical Immunology. 2010;**126**(6):1105-1118

[2] Nwaru BI et al. Prevalence of common food allergies in Europe: A systematic review and meta-analysis. Allergy. 2014;**69**(8):992-1007

[3] Prescott S, Allen KJ. Food allergy: Riding the second wave of the allergy epidemic. Pediatric Allergy and Immunology. 2011;**22**(2):155-160

[4] van der Hulst AE, Klip H, Brand PL. Risk of developing asthma in young children with atopic eczema: A systematic review. The Journal of Allergy and Clinical Immunology. 2007;**120**(3):565-569

[5] Thomsen SF. Epidemiology and natural history of atopic diseases. European Clinical Respiratory Journal. 2015;**2**. DOI: 10.3402/ecrj.v2.24642

[6] Belgrave DC et al. Atopic dermatitis and respiratory allergy: What is the link. Current Dermatology Reports. 2015;**4**(4):221-227. DOI: 10.1007/s13671-015-0121-6

[7] Goksor E et al. The allergic march comprises the coexistence of related patterns of allergic disease not just the progressive development of one disease. Acta Paediatrica. 2016;**105**(12):1472-1479. DOI: 10.1111/apa.13515

[8] Bingefors K et al. Self-reported lifetime prevalence of atopic dermatitis and co-morbidity with asthma and eczema in adulthood: A population-based cross-sectional survey. Acta Dermato-Venereologica. 2013;**93**(4):438-441. DOI: 10.2340/00015555-1522

[9] Paternoster L et al. Identification of atopic dermatitis subgroups in children from 2 longitudinal birth cohorts. The Journal of Allergy and Clinical Immunology. 2018;**141**(3):964-971

[10] Barker JN et al. Null mutations in the filaggrin gene (FLG) determine major susceptibility to early-onset atopic dermatitis that persists into adulthood. The Journal of Investigative Dermatology. 2007;**127**(3):564-567. DOI: 10.1038/sj.jid.5700587

[11] Margolis DJ et al. Thymic stromal lymphopoietin variation, filaggrin loss of function, and the persistence of atopic dermatitis. JAMA Dermatology. 2014;**150**(3):254-259. DOI: 10.1001/jamadermatol.2013.7954

[12] Ashley SE et al. The skin barrier function gene SPINK5 is associated with challenge-proven IgE-mediated food allergy in infants. Allergy. 2017;**72**(9):1356-1364. DOI: 10.1111/all.13143

[13] Marenholz I, Esparza-Gordillo J, Lee YA. The genetics of the skin barrier in eczema and other allergic disorders. Current Opinion in Allergy and Clinical Immunology. 2015;**15**(5):426-434. DOI: 10.1097/aci.0000000000000194

[14] Cianferoni A, Spergel J. The importance of TSLP in allergic disease and its role as a potential therapeutic target. Expert Review of Clinical Immunology. 2014;**10**(11):1463-1474. DOI: 10.1586/1744666x.2014.967684

[15] Czarnowicki T, Krueger JG, Guttman-Yassky E. Skin barrier and immune dysregulation in atopic dermatitis: An evolving story with important clinical implications. The Journal of Allergy and Clinical Immunology. In Practice. 2014;**2**(4):371-379. Quiz 380-1. DOI: 10.1016/j.jaip.2014.03.006

[16] Schleimer RP, Berdnikovs S. Etiology of epithelial barrier dysfunction in patients with type 2 inflammatory diseases. The Journal of Allergy and Clinical Immunology. 2017;**139**(6):1752-1761. DOI: 10.1016/j.jaci.2017.04.010

[17] Strid J et al. Disruption of the stratum corneum allows potent epicutaneous immunization with protein antigens resulting in a dominant systemic Th2 response. European Journal of Immunology. 2004;**34**(8):2100-2109. DOI: 10.1002/eji.200425196

[18] Spergel JM et al. Epicutaneous sensitization with protein antigen induces localized allergic dermatitis and hyperresponsiveness to methacholine after single exposure to aerosolized antigen in mice. The Journal of Clinical Investigation. 1998;**101**(8):1614-1622. DOI: 10.1172/jci1647

[19] Lack G et al. Factors associated with the development of peanut allergy in childhood. The New England Journal of Medicine. 2003;**348**(11):977-985. DOI: 10.1056/NEJMoa013536

[20] Fukutomi Y et al. Epidemiological link between wheat allergy and exposure to hydrolyzed wheat protein in facial soap. Allergy. 2014;**69**(10):1405-1411. DOI: 10.1111/all.12481

[21] Boussault P et al. Oat sensitization in children with atopic dermatitis: Prevalence, risks and associated factors. Allergy. 2007;**62**(11):1251-1256. DOI: 10.1111/j.1398-9995.2007.01527.x

[22] Saunes M et al. Early eczema and the risk of childhood asthma: A prospective, population-based study. BMC Pediatrics. 2012;**12**:168. DOI: 10.1186/1471-2431-12-168

[23] von Kobyletzki LB et al. Eczema in early childhood is strongly associated with the development of asthma and rhinitis in a prospective cohort. BMC Dermatology. 2012;**12**:11. DOI: 10.1186/1471-5945-12-11

[24] Gustafsson D, Sjoberg O, Foucard T. Development of allergies and asthma in infants and young children with atopic dermatitis--a prospective follow-up to 7 years of age. Allergy. 2000;**55**(3):240-245

[25] Tran MM et al. Predicting the atopic march: Results from the Canadian healthy infant longitudinal development study. The Journal of Allergy and Clinical Immunology. 2018;**141**(2):601-607.e8. DOI: 10.1016/j.jaci.2017.08.024

[26] Alduraywish SA et al. Is there a march from early food sensitization to later childhood allergic airway disease? Results from two prospective birth cohort studies. Pediatric Allergy and Immunology. 2017;**28**(1):30-37. DOI: 10.1111/pai.12651

[27] Hill DA et al. The epidemiologic characteristics of healthcare provider-diagnosed eczema, asthma, allergic rhinitis, and food allergy in children: A retrospective cohort study. BMC Pediatrics. 2016;**16**:133. DOI: 10.1186/s12887-016-0673-z

[28] Alduraywish SA et al. The march from early life food sensitization to allergic disease: A systematic review and meta-analyses of birth cohort studies. Allergy. 2016;**71**(1):77-89. DOI: 10.1111/all.12784

[29] Dunkin D, Berin MC, Mayer L. Allergic sensitization can be induced via multiple physiologic routes in an adjuvant-dependent manner. The Journal of Allergy and Clinical Immunology. 2011;**128**(6):1251-1258.e2. DOI: 10.1016/j.jaci.2011.06.007

[30] Liu AH. Revisiting the hygiene hypothesis for allergy and asthma. The Journal of Allergy and Clinical Immunology. 2015;**136**(4):860-865. DOI: 10.1016/j.jaci.2015.08.012

[31] Strachan DP. Hay fever, hygiene, and household size. British Medical Journal. 1989;**299**(6710):1259-1260

[32] Matricardi PM et al. Exposure to foodborne and orofecal microbes versus airborne viruses in relation to atopy and allergic asthma: Epidemiological study. British Medical Journal. 2000;**320**(7232):412-417

[33] Braun-Fahrlander C et al. Environmental exposure to endotoxin and its relation to asthma in school-age children. The New England Journal of Medicine. 2002;**347**(12):869-877. DOI: 10.1056/NEJMoa020057

[34] Ege MJ et al. Not all farming environments protect against the development of asthma and wheeze in children. The Journal of Allergy and Clinical Immunology. 2007;**119**(5):1140-1147. DOI: 10.1016/j.jaci.2007.01.037

[35] Rook GA. Review series on helminths, immune modulation and the hygiene hypothesis: The broader implications of the hygiene hypothesis. Immunology. 2009;**126**(1):3-11. DOI: 10.1111/j.1365-2567.2008.03007.x

[36] Blaser MJ, Falkow S. What are the consequences of the disappearing human microbiota? Nature Reviews. Microbiology. 2009;**7**(12):887-894. DOI: 10.1038/nrmicro2245

[37] Depner M et al. Bacterial microbiota of the upper respiratory tract and childhood asthma. The Journal of Allergy and Clinical Immunology. 2017;**139**(3):826-834.e13. DOI: 10.1016/j.jaci.2016.05.050

[38] Lodge CJ et al. Breastfeeding and asthma and allergies: A systematic review and meta-analysis. Acta Paediatrica. 2015;**104**(467):38-53. DOI: 10.1111/apa.13132

[39] Loss G et al. Consumption of unprocessed cow's milk protects infants from common respiratory infections. The Journal of Allergy and Clinical Immunology. 2015;**135**(1):56-62. DOI: 10.1016/j.jaci.2014.08.044

[40] Hasegawa K et al. Household siblings and nasal and fecal microbiota in infants. Pediatrics International. 2017;**59**(4):473-481. DOI: 10.1111/ped.13168

[41] Martin R et al. Early-life events, including mode of delivery and type of feeding, siblings and gender, shape the developing gut microbiota. PLoS One. 2016;**11**(6):e0158498. DOI: 10.1371/journal.pone.0158498

[42] Tun HM et al. Exposure to household furry pets influences the gut microbiota of infant at 3-4 months following various birth scenarios. Microbiome. 2017;**5**(1):40. DOI: 10.1186/s40168-017-0254-x

[43] Du Toit G et al. Food allergy: Update on prevention and tolerance. The Journal of Allergy and Clinical Immunology. 2018;**141**(1):30-40. DOI: 10.1016/j.jaci.2017.11.010

[44] Koplin JJ, Allen KJ. Optimal timing for solids introduction—Why are the guidelines always changing? Clinical and Experimental Allergy. 2013;**43**(8):826-834. DOI: 10.1111/cea.12090

[45] Perkin MR et al. Enquiring about tolerance (EAT) study: Feasibility of an early allergenic food introduction regimen. The Journal of Allergy and Clinical Immunology. 2016;**137**(5):1477-1486.e8. DOI: 10.1016/j.jaci.2015.12.1322

[46] Du Toit G et al. Randomized trial of peanut consumption in infants at risk for peanut allergy. The New England Journal of Medicine. 2015;**372**(9):803-813. DOI: 10.1056/NEJMoa1414850

[47] Du Toit G et al. Effect of avoidance on peanut allergy after early peanut

consumption. The New England Journal of Medicine. 2016;**374**(15):1435-1443. DOI: 10.1056/NEJMoa1514209

[48] Fewtrell M et al. Complementary feeding: A position paper by the European Society for Paediatric Gastroenterology, Hepatology, and Nutrition (ESPGHAN) committee on nutrition. Journal of Pediatric Gastroenterology and Nutrition. 2017;**64**(1):119-132. DOI: 10.1097/mpg.0000000000001454

[49] Muraro A et al. EAACI food allergy and anaphylaxis guidelines: Diagnosis and management of food allergy. Allergy. 2014;**69**(8):1008-1025. DOI: 10.1111/all.12429

[50] Molloy J et al. Is low vitamin D Status a risk factor for food allergy? Current evidence and future directions. Mini Reviews in Medicinal Chemistry. 2015;**15**(11):944-952

[51] Mullins RJ, Camargo CA. Latitude, sunlight, vitamin D, and childhood food allergy/anaphylaxis. Current Allergy and Asthma Reports. 2012;**12**(1):64-71. DOI: 10.1007/s11882-011-0230-7

[52] Allen KJ et al. Vitamin D insufficiency is associated with challenge-proven food allergy in infants. The Journal of Allergy and Clinical Immunology. 2013;**131**(4):1109-1116, 1116.e1-6. DOI: 10.1016/j.jaci.2013.01.017

[53] Litonjua AA. Vitamin D deficiency as a risk factor for childhood allergic disease and asthma. Current Opinion in Allergy and Clinical Immunology. 2012;**12**(2):179-185. DOI: 10.1097/ACI.0b013e3283507927

[54] Arshad SH et al. Early life risk factors for current wheeze, asthma, and bronchial hyperresponsiveness at 10 years of age. Chest. 2005;**127**(2):502-508

[55] Bergmann RL et al. Atopic dermatitis in early infancy predicts allergic airway disease at 5 years. Clinical and Experimental Allergy. 1998;**28**(8):965-970

[56] Bohme M et al. Atopic dermatitis and concomitant disease patterns in children up to two years of age. Acta Dermato-Venereologica. 2002;**82**(2):98-103

[57] Carlsten C et al. Atopic dermatitis in a high-risk cohort: Natural history, associated allergic outcomes, and risk factors. Annals of Allergy, Asthma and Immunology. 2013;**110**(1):24-28. DOI: 10.1016/j.anai.2012.10.005

[58] Klinnert MD et al. Onset and persistence of childhood asthma: Predictors from infancy. Pediatrics. 2001;**108**(4):E69

[59] Lowe AJ et al. Do boys do the atopic march while girls dawdle? The Journal of Allergy and Clinical Immunology. 2008;**121**(5):1190-1195

[60] Roduit C et al. Phenotypes of atopic dermatitis depending on the timing of onset and progression in childhood. JAMA Pediatrics. 2017;**171**(7):655-662

[61] Belgrave DC et al. Developmental profiles of eczema, wheeze, and rhinitis: Two population-based birth cohort studies. PLoS Medicine. 2014;**11**(10):e1001748

[62] Paller AS et al. The atopic march and atopic multimorbidity: Many trajectories, many pathways. The Journal of Allergy and Clinical Immunology. 2019;**143**(1):46-55. DOI: 10.1016/j.jaci.2018.11.006

[63] Campo P et al. Local allergic rhinitis: Implications for management. Clinical and Experimental Allergy. 2019;**49**(1):6-16. DOI: 10.1111/cea.13192

[64] Rondon C et al. Follow-up study in local allergic rhinitis shows a consistent entity not evolving to

systemic allergic rhinitis. The Journal of Allergy and Clinical Immunology. 2014;**133**(4):1026-1031. DOI: 10.1016/j.jaci.2013.10.034

[65] Sennekamp J et al. Local allergic nasal reactions convert to classic systemic allergic reactions: A long-term follow-up. International Archives of Allergy and Immunology. 2015;**166**(2):154-160. DOI: 10.1159/000380852

[66] Hatzler L et al. Molecular spreading and predictive value of preclinical IgE response to Phleum pratense in children with hay fever. The Journal of Allergy and Clinical Immunology. 2012;**130**(4):894-901.e5. DOI: 10.1016/j.jaci.2012.05.053

[67] Rondon C et al. Evolution of patients with nonallergic rhinitis supports conversion to allergic rhinitis. The Journal of Allergy and Clinical Immunology. 2009;**123**(5):1098-1102. DOI: 10.1016/j.jaci.2009.02.018

[68] Horimukai K et al. Application of moisturizer to neonates prevents development of atopic dermatitis. The Journal of Allergy and Clinical Immunology. 2014;**134**(4):824-830.e6. DOI: 10.1016/j.jaci.2014.07.060

[69] Lowe AJ et al. A randomized trial of a barrier lipid replacement strategy for the prevention of atopic dermatitis and allergic sensitization: The PEBBLES pilot study. The British Journal of Dermatology. 2018;**178**(1):e19-e21. DOI: 10.1111/bjd.15747

[70] Simpson EL et al. Emollient enhancement of the skin barrier from birth offers effective atopic dermatitis prevention. The Journal of Allergy and Clinical Immunology. 2014;**134**(4):818-823. DOI: 10.1016/j.jaci.2014.08.005

[71] Schneider L et al. Study of the atopic march: Development of atopic comorbidities. Pediatric Dermatology. 2016;**33**(4):388-398. DOI: 10.1111/pde.12867

[72] Stokholm J et al. Maturation of the gut microbiome and risk of asthma in childhood. Nature Communications. 2018;**9**(1):141. DOI: 10.1038/s41467-017-02573-2

[73] Myles IA et al. First-in-human topical microbiome transplantation with Roseomonas mucosa for atopic dermatitis. JCI Insight. 2018;**3**(9). DOI: 10.1172/jci.insight.120608

[74] Nakatsuji T et al. Antimicrobials from human skin commensal bacteria protect against *Staphylococcus aureus* and are deficient in atopic dermatitis. Science Translational Medicine. 2017;**9**(378). DOI: 10.1126/scitranslmed.aah4680

[75] Kalliomaki M et al. Probiotics in primary prevention of atopic disease: A randomised placebo-controlled trial. Lancet. 2001;**357**(9262):1076-1079. DOI: 10.1016/s0140-6736(00)04259-8

[76] Niccoli AA et al. Preliminary results on clinical effects of probiotic *Lactobacillus salivarius* LS01 in children affected by atopic dermatitis. Journal of Clinical Gastroenterology. 2014;**48**(Suppl 1):S34-S36. DOI: 10.1097/mcg.0000000000000233

[77] Cabana MD et al. Early probiotic supplementation for eczema and asthma prevention: A randomized controlled trial. Pediatrics. 2017;**140**(3). DOI: 10.1542/peds.2016-3000

[78] Zuccotti G et al. Probiotics for prevention of atopic diseases in infants: Systematic review and meta-analysis. Allergy. 2015;**70**(11):1356-1371. DOI: 10.1111/all.12700

[79] Cuello-Garcia CA et al. Probiotics for the prevention of allergy: A systematic review and meta-analysis of randomized controlled trials. The Journal of Allergy and Clinical

Immunology. 2015;**136**(4):952-961. DOI: 10.1016/j.jaci.2015.04.031

[80] Li L et al. Probiotic supplementation for prevention of atopic dermatitis in infants and children: A systematic review and meta-analysis. American Journal of Clinical Dermatology. 2018;**20**:367-377. DOI: 10.1007/s40257-018-0404-3

[81] Edwards MR et al. The potential of anti-infectives and immunomodulators as therapies for asthma and asthma exacerbations. Allergy. 2018;**73**(1): 50-63. DOI: 10.1111/all.13257

[82] Thomas DW, Greer FR. Probiotics and prebiotics in pediatrics. Pediatrics. 2010;**126**(6):1217-1231. DOI: 10.1542/peds.2010-2548

[83] Braegger C et al. Supplementation of infant formula with probiotics and/or prebiotics: A systematic review and comment by the ESPGHAN committee on nutrition. Journal of Pediatric Gastroenterology and Nutrition. 2011;**52**(2):238-250. DOI: 10.1097/MPG.0b013e3181fb9e80

[84] Fiocchi A et al. World Allergy Organization-McMaster University guidelines for allergic disease prevention (GLAD-P): Probiotics. World Allergy Organization Journal. 2015;**8**(1):4. DOI: 10.1186/s40413-015-0055-2

[85] Ownby DR, Johnson CC, Peterson EL. Exposure to dogs and cats in the first year of life and risk of allergic sensitization at 6 to 7 years of age. JAMA. 2002;**288**(8):963-972

[86] Bunyavanich S et al. Prenatal, perinatal, and childhood vitamin D exposure and their association with childhood allergic rhinitis and allergic sensitization. The Journal of Allergy and Clinical Immunology. 2016;**137**(4):1063-1070.e2. DOI: 10.1016/j.jaci.2015.11.031

[87] Yepes-Nunez JJ et al. Vitamin D supplementation in primary allergy prevention: Systematic review of randomized and non-randomized studies. Allergy. 2018;**73**(1):37-49. DOI: 10.1111/all.13241

[88] Iikura Y et al. Prevention of asthma by ketotifen in infants with atopic dermatitis. Annals of Allergy. 1992;**68**(3):233-236

[89] Wahn PU. Allergic factors associated with the development of asthma and the influence of cetirizine in a double-blind, randomised, placebo-controlled trial: First results of ETAC. Early Treatment of the Atopic Child. Pediatric Allergy and Immunology. 1998;**9**(3):116-124

[90] Zolkipli Z et al. Randomized controlled trial of primary prevention of atopy using house dust mite allergen oral immunotherapy in early childhood. The Journal of Allergy and Clinical Immunology. 2015;**136**(6):1541-1547.e11. DOI: 10.1016/j.jaci.2015.04.045

[91] Valovirta E et al. Results from the 5-year SQ grass sublingual immunotherapy tablet asthma prevention (GAP) trial in children with grass pollen allergy. The Journal of Allergy and Clinical Immunology. 2018;**141**(2):529-538.e13. DOI: 10.1016/j.jaci.2017.06.014

[92] Halken S et al. EAACI guidelines on allergen immunotherapy: Prevention of allergy. Pediatric Allergy and Immunology. 2017;**28**(8):728-745. DOI: 10.1111/pai.12807

[93] Kristiansen M et al. Allergen immunotherapy for the prevention of allergy: A systematic review and meta-analysis. Pediatric Allergy and Immunology. 2017;**28**(1):18-29. DOI: 10.1111/pai.12661

Chapter 2

Local Allergic Rhinitis: An Old Story but a New Entity

Ramit Maoz-Segal, Diti Machnes-Maayan, Irena Veksler-Offengenden, Shirly Frizinsky, Soad Hajyahia and Nancy Agmon-Levin

Abstract

Local allergic rhinitis (LAR) is a novel concept defining clinical allergic rhinitis with no evidence of systemic sensitization to aeroallergens. In this unique condition, the allergic response is confined to the nasal mucosa and can be demonstrated using different methods such as the immunoglobulin-E (IgE) level in the nasal secretions, nasal provocation test (NPT), or basophil activation test (BAT) with specific allergens or more sophisticated molecular diagnostic techniques. Furthermore, local allergic rhinitis can be relieved by interventions used to treat systemic allergic conditions such as antihistamines or anti-IgE monoclonal antibodies. Last but not least, several small studies demonstrated the efficacy of allergen immunotherapy for ameliorating LAR symptoms. In this chapter we reviewed old data and new concepts regarding clinical manifestation, plausible mechanisms, and treatments of LAR. The long-standing question whether LAR is an integral part of the "atopic spectrum" or it is a single-organ immune-mediated disease, is yet to be determined.

Keywords: allergic rhinitis, local allergic rhinitis, mite, rhinitis, immunotherapy

1. Definition of local allergic rhinitis

Local allergic rhinitis (LAR) is defined by symptoms suggestive of allergic rhinitis (AR), but with no detected sensitivity to an allergen using common allergy testing, while allergen-specific immunoglobulin-E (IgE) in the nasal mucosa can be detected.

2. Background

The first report of local production of IgE in the nasal mucosa was documented in 1975 among patients with typical symptoms of allergic rhinitis and negative allergy evaluation (i.e., negative skin prick tests (SPT) or serum-specific IgE (sIgE)). In this early report, specific IgE antibodies to *Dermatophagoides pteronyssinus* (house dust mite) had been detected in the nasal secretions of patients [1]. Later on, several methods to detect IgE in nasal secretions were evaluated, but only in 1989 a direct measuring technique was established [2]. This was tracked in

IntechOpen

2010, by defining the concept *entopy* as opposed to atopy. Although still somewhat controversial, *entopy* addresses local production of IgE in the nasal and respiratory mucosa, while atopy is characterized by serum-specific IgE and positive skin reaction [3, 4]. In recent years advances in documentation of nasal IgE production among patients with typical symptoms of allergic rhinitis substantiated the entity of LAR, which is now accepted and relevant worldwide.

3. Prevalence

The prevalence of LAR is uncertain and was long considered a rare disorder. In recent years, with the improvement of diagnostic methods, new and surprising data has emerged. In 2012 Rondon et al. reported a prevalence of 25.7% of LAR among a group of 428 adult patients with chronic rhinitis. In the same cohort, 63.1% were diagnosed with AR and 11.2% with non-allergic rhinitis (NAR). The most frequently causative allergen in both LAR and AR was *D. pteronyssinus* (*house dust mite*) [4]. Similar ratio between LAR and AR was reported by Bozek et al. among 219 elderly patients (mean age 65.8 years). The prevalence of LAR was 21% and that of AR was 40.2%, and *again D. pteronyssinus* was found to be the major culprit allergen [5]. However, this data was obtained in selected populations of patients with chronic rhinitis, while the prevalence of LAR in the general population is yet to be established.

4. Diagnosis of LAR

As mentioned above, LAR has to be considered in the differential diagnosis of AR, when no evidence of systemic atopy is present. The evaluation of a patient suspected to have LAR should include a detailed clinical history, typically resembling AR, as well as assessment of comorbidities, such as ocular, skin, and bronchial symptoms. This may enable further evaluation for systemic atopy or a filter for patients with non-allergic rhinitis (NAR; see **Table 1**). A detailed physical examination includes inspection of the nasal cavity via nasal endoscopy, and for some patients, a CT scan may be required to exclude other causes of chronic rhinitis. This should be followed by tests to verify sensitization to aeroallergens, either skin prick tests (SPT) or serum-specific IgE. It has been suggested that when there is a high index of suspicion of allergy and no reaction to SPT, intradermal skin tests to common aeroallergens may be considered. In the absence of evidence for systemic sensitization, one must prove local rhino-mucosa hyper-reactivity to aeroallergens in order to diagnose LAR [6, 7] (**Figure 1**). Three methods can be used to diagnose LAR:

1. *Nasal allergen provocation test* (*NAPT*) is considered the gold standard for LAR diagnosis. NAPT consists of eliciting a local nasal allergic response by exposure to allergens. A response is characterized by rhinorrhea, itching, sneezing, edema of the nasal mucosa, and increased airflow resistance following exposure of the nasal mucosa to a specific allergen. NAPT has the potential to differentiate between allergic (both AR and LAR) and the non-allergic rhinitis (NAR) or healthy controls. Furthermore, among allergic patients it could differentiate between clinically relevant and nonrelevant allergen sensitizations. NAPT could be done with single allergen or with multiple aeroallergens in one session [8]. In another study 60% of LAR patients responded immediately to nasal allergen provocation test (NAPT) with a specific allergen demonstrating

nasal symptoms, elevated tryptase (mast cell activation marker), and eosinophil cationic protein (ECP marker of eosinophil activation) [9, 10]. Notably, this method may highlight a subgroup of patients that suffers from both local and systemic sensitizations, namely, the "dual allergic rhinitis (DAR)" patient. For instance, a DAR patient may suffer from perennial symptoms, but his allergy testing will demonstrate sensitivity only to seasonal allergens, whereas his NAPT study will be positive to perennial allergens.

NAPT is a sensitive and specific technique, although it requires special training and is time-consuming [8]. Furthermore, it has some pitfalls. Nasal challenge with saline prior to NAPT is recommended to rule out non-specific nasal hyper-reactivity, which may induce a false-positive result. Having said that, there is yet lack of standardization regarding allergenic extract, dose, timing, and outcome definitions of NAPT [9].

2. *sIgE in the nasal secretions* is determined in nasal lavage fluid (e.g., after natural exposure), after NAPT, or following mucosal brushing [10]. Notably, sIgE could also be measured in nasal biopsies for more accurate results, but in the clinical practice, noninvasive methods might be preferable. The measurement of sIgE in nasal secretions is dependent on the technique used. Thus, although positive results are highly specific (>90%), sensitivity is rather low utilizing nasal lavage, ranging from 22 to 40%, most likely owing to dilution effect [7, 9]. Hence, when the lavage results are negative and there is a high index of suspicion, it is recommended to perform a more invasive procedure, as specified earlier.

3. *Basophil activation test* (*BAT*): Peripheral basophils are key cells in allergic responses and are involved in immediate IgE-mediated reactions. Their primary role is to degranulate pro-inflammatory mediators following stimulation and activation by allergens. Basophil activation can be measured by flow

- Chronic rhinosinusitis
    - With nasal polyposis (CRSWNP)
    - Without nasal polyposis (CRSW/ONP)
- Non-allergic rhinitis
    - Drug-related
    - Hormonal
    - Related to systemic diseases:
        1. Genetic disease: cystic fibrosis, primary ciliary dyskinesia
        2. Autoimmune/inflammatory diseases: granulomatosis, relapsing polychondritis, sarcoidosis
        3. Amyloidosis
        4. Malignancy related
    - Atrophic rhinitis
    - Occupational rhinitis (irritant)
    - Rhinitis medicamentosa
    - Anatomic defects:
        1. Local: Septal deviation, turbinate hypertrophy, adenoid hypertrophy (nonatopic variant)
        2. Nonlocal: Cerebrospinal fluid leaking

Table 1.
Differential diagnosis of allergic and local allergic rhinitis.

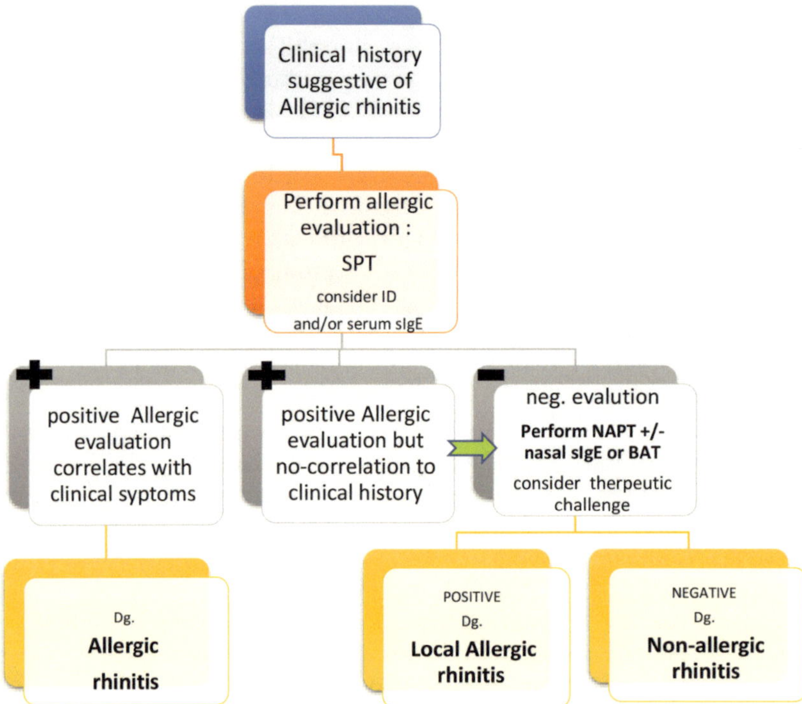

Figure 1.
Allergic rhinitis diagnostic algorithm. SPT, skin prick test; ID, intradermal skin tests; sIgE, specific IgE; NAPT, nasal provocation test; BAT, basophil activation test.

cytometry in which surface activation markers such as CD63 are quantified. The BAT is a flow cytometry-based assay performed on patient's peripheral blood, where the expression of these activation markers is measured following stimulation with allergen. BAT have been extensively studied and validated for in vitro diagnosis of sensitization to inhalant and food allergens, Hymenoptera venom, and several drug hypersensitivities [11]. The first evidence of specific basophil activation in peripheral blood from patients with LAR was reported in 2013 by Gome et al. [12], in which it was demonstrated for the first time that the activation of basophils in LAR patients was mediated by specific IgE to *D. pteronyssinus*. BAT was linked with 50% sensitivity and >90% specificity, which may be superior to the current data on sIgE in nasal lavage (e.g., specificity of 22%). In another study of patients with LAR to *Olea europaea*, BAT sensitivity was 66% with >90% specificity [7].

In summary, BAT has a medium-grade sensitivity and a high specificity for the diagnosis of local sIgE, which may outperform other methods for sIgE detection. It is less time-consuming; however, it is performer dependent compared to NAPT.

5. The pathophysiology of LAR

The pathogenesis of allergic rhinitis (AR) is well established. It is a Th2-mediated disease which involves mast cell activation, recruitment of eosinophils, basophils and T cells expressing Th2 cytokines, and secretion of interleukin as

IL-4, IL-13, IL-5, and others. The pathophysiology of LAR is less well established, and the question why the majority of allergic patients exhibit systemic sensitization (atopy) while some develop only local responses (entopy) is yet to be answered. Nonetheless, it has been suggested that the natural history of allergy is composed of multiple steps leading eventually to atopy. In a recent review, Dullaers et al. [13] suggested that the first step to atopy takes place in the nasal mucosa, where allergen-specific IgE is produced. The authors further hypothesized that some subjects lack spillover of these mucosal-produced allergen-specific IgEs into the circulation. In another study, the detection of allergen-specific IgE on the surfaces of peripheral basophils from patients with LAR eluded to the idea that the second step to atopy is on the surface of peripheral basophils and other target immune cells, followed by the third and final step which is the detection of serum-specific IgE and skin mast cell sensitization [12]. Thus, differences between LAR and AR may explain different stages of sensitization to allergen. For example, it was demonstrated that following nasal provocation of patients allergic to olive, the ECP levels in nasal lavage were significantly higher in both AR and LAR patients than in controls, while basophil activation test (BAT) was higher only in the LAR group, which potentially represents an earlier step in sensitization, associated more closely with LAR [14].

In contrast, similarities between AR and LAR pathophysiology were observed while evaluating the immunologic responses to therapy and particularly to immunotherapy. Namely, alike AR patients a significant increase of serum-specific IgG4 antibodies is observed following allergen immunotherapy among LAR patients. This not only substantiates the IgE-mediated mechanism of disease but also the notion that LAR may be the prodrome of AR [15]. Last but not least, allergen-specific IgEs to various allergens in the nasal scrapings from patients with AR, non-allergic rhinitis (NAR), and healthy controls were reported to be 86.7, 33.3, and 50%, respectively. Thus, although a wide difference between allergic and non-allergic patients was documented, a relatively high percent of IgE production was observed among controls [16]. One may suggest that healthy controls were sensitized but developed spontaneous tolerance, e.g., “a backward step” following the first, second, or third stage of atopy.

6. Local allergic rhinitis and comorbidity

AR is an essential part of the “atopic march” [17] and thereby associated with comorbidities, such as asthma, atopic dermatitis, food allergies eosinophilic esophagitis, allergic conjunctivitis, chronic rhinosinusitis with nasal polyposis (CRSwNP), and more [18]. The association of these comorbidities with local allergic rhinitis (LAR) was less explored [19], although bronchial symptoms have been reported in patients with LAR [20] and any chronic rhinitis is a risk factor for poorly controlled asthma with recurrent hospital visits [19]. Recently, self-reported bronchial symptoms, suggestive of asthma, were reported in over 30% of patients with LAR, suggesting a new asthma phenotype, “local allergic asthma” [21, 22]. As in classical allergic rhinitis, conjunctival symptoms were also associated with LAR. It was shown that patients with LAR experience ocular symptoms during nasal exacerbations due to allergen exposure or during in vitro nasal provocation tests [20]. In one study, this was the most prevalent comorbidity associated with LAR [23]. In a recent study by Rondon et al. [19], a 10-year follow-up of 176 LAR patients entailed other comorbidities, such as food allergy and drug hypersensitivity, which were documented only in few patients.

7. Treatment of LAR

In daily practice NAPT, BAT, or other specific tests are rarely performed. Hence, performing a therapeutic trial with antihistamines may be beneficial for diagnosis of LAR. Early and substantial response to antihistamine further supports an allergic histamine-driven mechanism. In the same line of thought, treatment with nasal corticosteroid spray may be clinically beneficial, but will not enable to differentiate causes of chronic rhinitis. Most LAR patients are currently treated similarly to AR patients, and according to the allergic rhinitis and its impact on asthma (ARIA) guidelines. This is done by using personal and environmental education, allergen avoidance measures and non-specific pharmacologic modalities, such as, intranasal corticosteroids, and oral and intranasal antihistamines [7–10]. Having said that, such non-specific therapy for LAR will ameliorate symptoms but alike AR will not change the natural progression of disease.

Immunotherapy is a common therapeutic modality for moderate to severe unresponsive AR. Allergen immunotherapy is based on gradual exposure to a culprit allergen via subcutaneous or sublingual exposure. This will eventually result in "induced tolerance" to the targeted allergen and amelioration of the allergic response. Allergen immunotherapy is highly effective and safe and confers long-term clinical benefit in adequately selected patients. Furthermore, it is the only etiological treatment for AR and asthma which conveys disease-modifying effect that can actually change the natural course of the disease [8, 9]. Thus, although LAR is by definition a local rather than systemic disease, few studies provide evidence for clinical benefit of allergen immunotherapy among LAR patients. These studies demonstrated a significant symptom improvement, an increase in the number of medication free days, and a beneficial effect on ocular symptoms, asthma control, and quality of life compared to placebo, as well as tolerance induction defined by an increase in allergen-specific IgG4 [6–8, 10].

8. Conclusions

In the last decade, growing evidence indicates that nasal reactivity to aeroallergens can occur in the absence of evidence of systemic atopy. The published literature raised the suspicion that many patients diagnosed previously as suffering from non-allergic rhinitis actually suffer from LAR. This may be of importance as treatment options differ between non-allergic and AR/LAR diseases. Diagnosis of LAR remains a challenge, as none of the diagnostic methods suggested are optimal nor commonly available in most centers. Therefore, high index of suspicion, utilizing specific methods if accessible as well as therapeutic challenge, may enable correct and early diagnosis. This may enable specific allergen-directed interventions (e.g., allergen immunotherapy), as well as early detection and treatment of comorbidities (like asthma and conjunctivitis). In this regard, implementation of NAPT, BAT, and other methods of diagnosis, especially in referral centers, as well as long-term studies to better define the mechanisms, course, and response to therapy of LAR, is needed.

Author details

Ramit Maoz-Segal[1†], Diti Machnes-Maayan[1,2†], Irena Veksler-Offengenden[1], Shirly Frizinsky[1], Soad Hajyahia[1,2] and Nancy Agmon-Levin[1,2*]

1 Clinical Immunology, Angioedema and Allergy Unit, Center for Autoimmune Diseases, Sheba Medical Center, Tel Hashomer, Israel

2 Sackler School of Medicine, Tel Aviv University, Ramat-Aviv, Israel

*Address all correspondence to: nancy.agmon-levin@sheba.health.gov.il

†Equally contributed

References

[1] Huggings KG, Brostoff J. Local production of specific IgE antibodies in allergic-rhinitis patients with negative skin tests. Lancet. 1975;**2**(7926):148-150

[2] Marcucci F, Sensi L. A new method for IgE detection in nasal mucosa. Clinical and Experimental Allergy. 1989;**19**(2):157-162

[3] Forester JP, Calabria CW. Local production of IgE in the respiratory mucosa and the concept of entopy: Does allergy exist in nonallergic rhinitis. Annals of Allergy, Asthma & Immunology. 2010;**105**(4):249-255

[4] Rondón C, Campo P, Galindo L, Blanca-López N, Cassinello MS, Rodriguez-Bada JL, et al. Prevalence and clinical relevance of local allergic rhinitis. Allergy. 2012;**67**(10):1282-1288

[5] Bozek A, Ignasiak B, Kasperska-Zajac A, Scierski W, Grzanka A, Jarzab J. Local allergic rhinitis in elderly patients. Annals of Allergy, Asthma & Immunology. 2015;**114**(3):199-2012

[6] Fokkens WJ. More papers, more issues. Rhinology. 2019;**57**(1):1

[7] Campo P, Eguiluz-Gracia I, Bogas G, Salas M, Plaza Serón C, Pérez N, et al. Local allergic rhinitis: Implications for management. Clinical and Experimental Allergy. 2019;**49**:6-16

[8] Campo P, Salas M, Blanca-López N, Rondón C. Local allergic rhinitis. Immunology and Allergy Clinics of North America. 2016;**36**:321-332

[9] Arasi S, Pajno GB, Lau S, Matricardi PM. Local allergic rhinitis: A critical reappraisal from a pediatric perspective. Pediatric Allergy and Immunology. 2016;**27**:569-573

[10] Altıntoprak N, Kar M, Muluk NB, Oktemer T, Ipci K, Birdane L, et al. Update on local allergic rhinitis. International Journal of Pediatric Otorhinolaryngology. 2016;**87**:105-109

[11] Kleine-Tebbe J, Erdmann S, Knol EF, MacGlashan DW, Poulsen LK, Gibbs BF. Diagnostic tests based on human basophils: Potentials, pitfalls and perspectives. International Archives of Allergy and Immunology. 2006;**141**:79-90

[12] Gomez E, Campo P, Rondon C, Barrionuevo E, Blanca-Lopez N, Torres MJ, et al. Role of the basophil activation test in the diagnosis of local allergic rhinitis. The Journal of Allergy and Clinical Immunology. 2013;**132**(4):975-976

[13] Dullaers M, De Bruyne R, Ramadani F, Gould HJ, Geavert P, Lambrecht BN. The who, where and when of IgE in allergic airway disease. The Journal of Allergy and Clinical Immunology. 2012;**129**:635-645

[14] Gelardi M, Guglielmi AV, Iannuzzi L, Quaranta VN, Quaranta N, Landi M, et al. Local allergic rhinitis: Entopy or spontaneous response? World Allergy Organization Journal. 2016;**9**(1):39

[15] Campo P, Villalba M, Barrionuevo E, Rondon C, Salas M, Galindo L, et al. Immunologic responses to the major allergen of *Olea europaea* in local and systemic allergic rhinitis subjects. Clinical and Experimental Allergy. 2015;**45**(11):1703-1712

[16] Ebo DG, Bridts CH, Hagendorens MM, Aerts NE, De Clerck LS, Stevens WJ. Basophil activation test by flow cytometry: Present and future applications in allergology. Cytometry. Part B, Clinical Cytometry. 2008;**74**(4):201-210

[17] Tsilochristou OA, Douladiris N, Makris M, Papadopoulos NG. Pediatric

allergic rhinitis and asthma: Can the march be halted? Paediatric Drugs. 2013;**15**(6):431-440

[18] Cingi P, Gevaert R, Mösges C, Rondon V, Hox M, Rudenko NB, et al. Multi-morbidities of allergic rhinitis in adults: European academy of allergy and clinical immunology task force report. Clinical and Translational Allergy. 2017;**7**:17

[19] Rondon C, Campo P, Eguiluz-Gracia I, et al. Local allergic rhinitis is an independent rhinitis phenotype: The results of a 10-year follow-up study. Allergy. 2017;**73**:470-478

[20] Rondon C, Campo P, Galindo L, Blanca-López N, Cassinello MS, Rodriguez-Bada JL, et al. Prevalence and clinical relevance of local allergic rhinitis. Allergy. 2012;**67**(10):1282-1288

[21] Rondon C, Campo P, Salas M, Aranda A, Molina A, Gonzalez M, et al. Efficacy and safety of *D. pteronyssinus* immunotherapy in local allergic rhinitis: A double-blind placebo-con- trolled clinical trial. Allergy. 2016;**71**(7):1057-1061

[22] Campo P, Eguiluz-Gracia I, Plaza-Seron MC, Salas M, Rodríguez MJ, Pérez-Sánchez N, et al. Bronchial asthma triggered by house dust mites in patients with local allergic rhinitis. Allergy. 2019. [Epub ahead of print]

[23] Rondon C, Campo P, Zambonino MA, Blanca-Lopez N, Torres MG, Melendez L, et al. Follow-up study in local allergic rhinitis shows a consistent entity not evolving to systemic allergic rhinitis. The Journal of Allergy and Clinical Immunology. 2014;**133**:1026-1031

Section 2

Sinusitis

Chapter 3

Use of Nasal Cytology in Diagnosis of Sinonasal Disorders

Marco Capelli

Abstract

Nasal cytology is an important diagnostic tool in nasal disorders, especially those regarding nasal mucosa. This technique allows clinicians to observe the morphology and the structure of nasal epithelium cells—such as ciliated, mucous-secreting, striated, and basal cells—and to detect the presence of degenerative or phlogistic phenomena in the respiratory epithelium. Moreover, it makes it easy to identify the presence of inflammatory cells, such as neutrophils, eosinophils, and mast cell. Over the past few years, nasal cytology allowed researchers to discover new clinical issues that were still unexplored: the nonallergic rhinitis with eosinophils, the nonallergic rhinitis with mast cells, the nonallergic rhinitis with neutrophils, and the nonallergic rhinitis with eosinophils and mast cells. Nasal cytology is easy to perform and barely invasive; therefore, it can easily be repeated. Since it makes it possible to evaluate the patient's response to a therapy, the technique is a very useful tool in follow-up checks of nasal disorders. We have reported in the following chapter our working experience, and we observed the results of cytological exams performed in our Center from 2013 to 2018. We therefore developed an easy and intuitive classification of sinonasal chronic inflammatory diseases.

Keywords: nasal cytology, rhinosinusitis, neutrophils, eosinophils, classification

1. Introduction

The nose is composed of two nasal cavities separated by an osteocartilaginous structure called nasal septum. The initial portion is called nasal vestibule, while the next part is called nasal cavity. The nasal cavity borders on the nasopharynx, from which it is separated by the choanae. In the most cranial portion of the nasal fossa, we find the olfactory fissure. This region is responsible for the perception of odorous stimuli. The nasal cavities are occupied by osseous structures with mucous lining called turbinates. These are divided as follows: the inferior turbinate that through its cavernous vascular tissue contributes to humidify and heat the inspired air, the middle turbinate that anatomically defines a sort of pre-sinus space, and at last the superior turbinate. In some cases we also recognize a fourth turbinate called supreme [1].

We observe four different nasal epithelia. A layered keratinized floor epithelium covers the region of the nasal vestibule, and an epithelium called transitional is located at the level of the valve. On the other hand, the nasal cavities are covered by a mucosa with pseudostratified ciliated epithelium (enriched with olfactory cells at the level of the olfactory fissure). The ciliated pseudostratified epithelium is composed of four types of cells: ciliated cells, muciparous cells, columnar cells, and basal cells, anchored by desmosomes and hemidesmosomes. This epithelium is separated from

IntechOpen

the underlying tonaca propria by a basal membrane. In the context of the tonaca propria, we can find three layers. At the beginning, just below the basement membrane, we can find the lymphoid layer, which is characterized by the richness of lymphocytes (nasal-associated lymphoid tissue (NALT)). Then we have the glandular layer, characterized by glands that have a significant immune function producing secretions rich in lysozyme and IgA. Last, we can find the vascular layer, characterized by important vascular representation, especially in the mucosa of the inferior turbinate [2].

This brief description of microscopic anatomy of the nasal mucosa allows us to highlight the many important physiological functions it performs.

First of all, in the respiratory epithelium, the mucociliary clearing action is carried out thanks to the cooperation of ciliated and muciparous cells. This process is fundamental in determining the circulation of mucus, and therefore it performs a nasal cleaning with immuno-protective tasks [3]. At the level of the superficial mucous layer (thanks to the presence of lymphatic tissue) and at the level of the intermediate glandular layer (thanks to the secretion of lysozyme and IgA), immunocompetence functions are also performed. At last, the vascular layer, thanks to the presence of cavernous tissue, allows to change the physical-chemical characteristics of the air inhaled before its passage in the middle and lower respiratory tract [2]. With the passage of air through the nasal cavities, water vapor is transferred through the mucosa of the inferior turbinates with consequent lowering of oxygen partial pressures [4]. Furthermore, due to the contact between the mucosal surface of the turbinate and the air, the heating of the same is ensured [5].

The pathology of the rhinosinusal district appears to be varied and diversified [2], and it is characterized by many different types of clinical entities that sometimes are present individually, sometimes they overlap: this creates, in our opinion, classification difficulties. Another critical aspect for clinicians is to understand the real extent of rhinosinus disease, that is, if we are dealing with an exclusively nasal or sinus involvement or an involvement of both districts.

Our experience has led us to use in diagnosis of a rhinosinusopathy both a cytological examination of the nasal mucosa that will allow us to identify the problem and a radiological study (better if using cone beam CT) to define the real extent of the problem.

In this discussion we will explain how to perform a cytological examination and how to interpret it, and we will try to define a systematic classification of rhinopathies relying on the analysis of cytological compartments of patients affected by rhinopathy from our Center in the last 5 years.

2. Materials and methods

For about 10 years, we have been analyzing cytological samples from the lower turbinate mucosa in patients with chronic rhinopathies. This type of evaluation allowed us to study the microscopic characteristics of the healthy nasal mucosa and to identify the characteristic aspects of the different forms of rhinopathy. Performing a cytological examination is simple, rapid, and minimally invasive. It is also a cost-effective investigation.

From October 2013 to September 2018, we performed cytological sampling and subsequent microscopic analysis on the sample obtained from 300 patients with chronic rhinopathy. These patients reported suffering from several months or even years of nasal respiratory obstruction, rhinorrhea, in some cases complaining of recurrent headache or hyposmia or sneezing and nasal itching.

The cytological examination of each patient was performed according to the Italian Academy of Nasal Cytology (AICNA) procedures. We briefly summarized the modalities in the following paragraph.

2.1 How to perform a cytological sampling

2.1.1 Sampling

Through a small spoon called Rhino-Probe®, we collect mucous material joined to cells of the nasal mucosa, exerting a slight pressure on the body of the inferior turbinate. This technique is called nasal scraping (there are other sampling techniques such as brushing, nasal swab, and the washing that we report but of which we have no experience).

2.1.2 Processing

The material taken is distributed on a special slide, while avoiding to touch the surface of the slide with your fingers while always using gloves.

2.1.3 Fixation and coloring

We proceed to fix the material taken on the slide, then we apply the May-Grunwald-Giemsa (MGG) coloration. In our experience, we have been using a fast-acting MGG staining method (MGG Quick Stain®) for some years now. Cytological staining method is very numerous and each of them has its own specificity and application. In nasal cytology the most widely used is the MGG method which is able to easily differentiate the various cells found in the nasal mucosa.

2.1.4 Assembly of the slide

Through a specific synthetic product (Bio Mount HM®) the cover slip is applied above the slide. This way, the sample is ready to be observed.

2.2 Microscopic observation

The analysis of the sample of cytology material mounted on the slide is done with an optical microscope equipped with multiple objectives, each with different magnification power.

Phenotype	Cellularity	Sublcasses
Cellular	Neutrophil	
	Eosninofil	
	Mast cell	
	Miscellaneous	Neutrophil-eosinophil
		Neutrophil-mast cellular
		Neutro-eosino-masto cellular
		Eosinophil-mast cellular
Non cellular	Medicamentosa	
	Hormonal	
	From decubitus	
	Atrophic	
	Mechanical	

Table 1.
Classification of rhinosinusitis.

Initially, a general inspection of the material is carried out with a lower magnification objective (4×/0.10). Once the most significant part of the sample has been identified, the evaluation will be carried out with increasingly powerful objectives to exploit the maximum possible magnification (100×/1.25) with the help of oil for immersion.

In accordance with the guidelines of the Italian Academy of Nasal Cytology (AICNA), for each sample taken, we analyze at least 50 fields at maximum magnification (100×/25) by counting the different types of cells found. The observed data are then shown in a **Table 1**.

3. Results

We have collected in **Figure 1** the results of the cytological tests performed from October 2013 to September 2018 (**Figure 1**).

Of the 300 patients studied, 154 (equal to 53.66%) were affected by a pathology of the nasal mucosa of neutrophilic type that is characterized by the presence of more or less numerous neutrophil granulocytes. The majority of them, 136 patients (88.31%), had chronic nonpolyposis pathology, while only 18 (11.69%) of them presented a polyposis pathology (**Figure 2**). The patients with nonpolyposis pathology were subjected to cone beam computed tomography (CBCT). Ninety-seven patients (71.32%) showed a pathological thickening of the paranasal sinuses mucosa. This situation indicates an involvement of the paranasal sinuses by the pathology and suggests a diagnosis of chronic rhinosinusitis (**Figure 3**).

Thirty-four patients, equal to 11.85% of the total, showed a significant presence in the nasal mucosa of eosinophilic granulocytes. Of these, 29.41% of patients (10) had polyposis, while 70.59% of patients (24) had nonpolyposis (**Figure 4**).

Only five patients (1.74% of the total) showed instead a significant presence of mast cells in the nasal mucosa, and in no case we observed a form of polyposis. Finally, 32.75% of patients (94) had a mixed cell infiltration in the samples of nasal mucosa (**Figure 1**). Of these, 23.40% (22 patients) presented a polyposis pathology (**Figure 5**).

We analyzed the cytotypes of the "mixed cellularity rhinosinusopathy" category, distinguishing four subclasses: neutrophil-eosinophil forms (50 patients, equal to 53.19%), neutrophil-mast cell forms (8 patients equal to 8.51%),

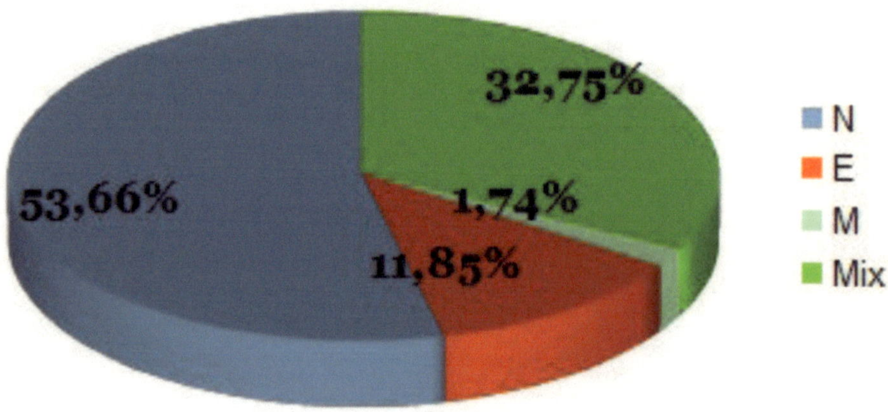

Figure 1.
Type of cells in nasal pathology.

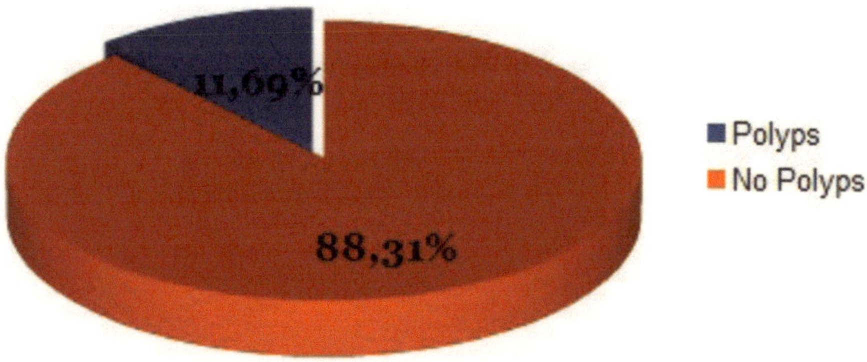

Figure 2.
Neutrophil pathology: presence of polyps.

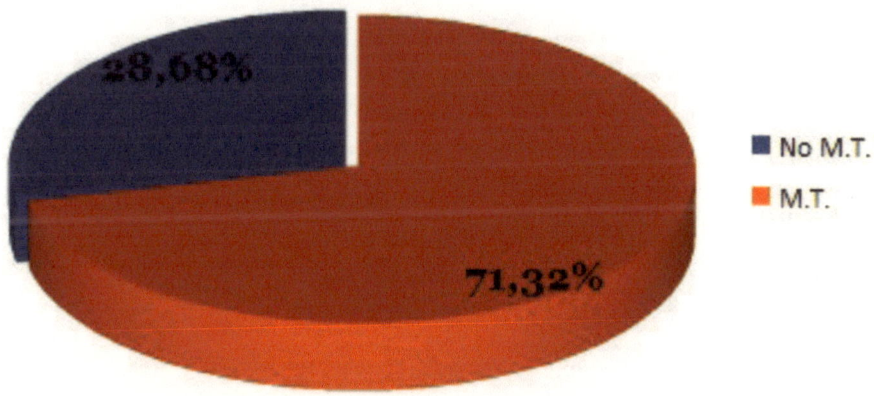

Figure 3.
Neutrophil nonpolypoid pathology: mucosal thickening.

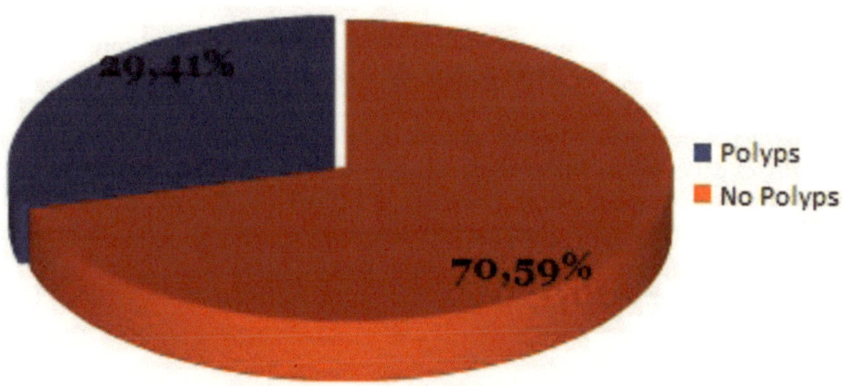

Figure 4.
Eosinophil pathology: presence of polyps.

neutrophil-eosinophil-mastocyte forms (24 patients equal to 25.53%), and eosinophil-mast cell forms (12 patients equal to 12.77%) as indicated in **Figure 6**.

In 33 patients (equal to 11% of the total patients studied), we did not find any pathological changes in the nasal mucosa.

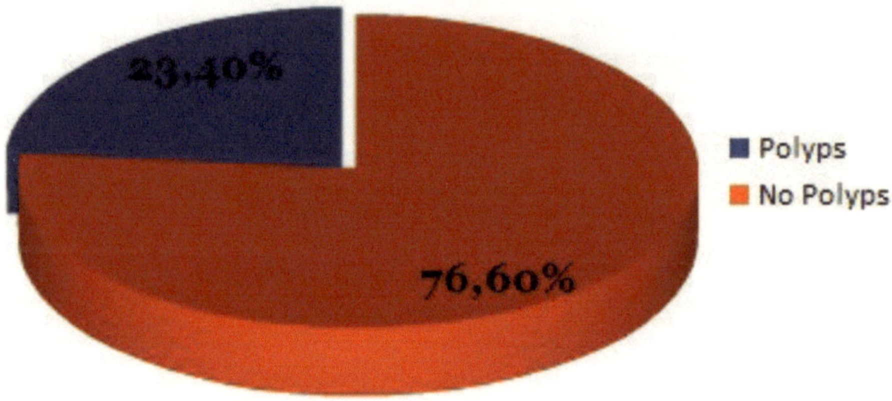

Figure 5.
Mixed pathology: presence of polyps.

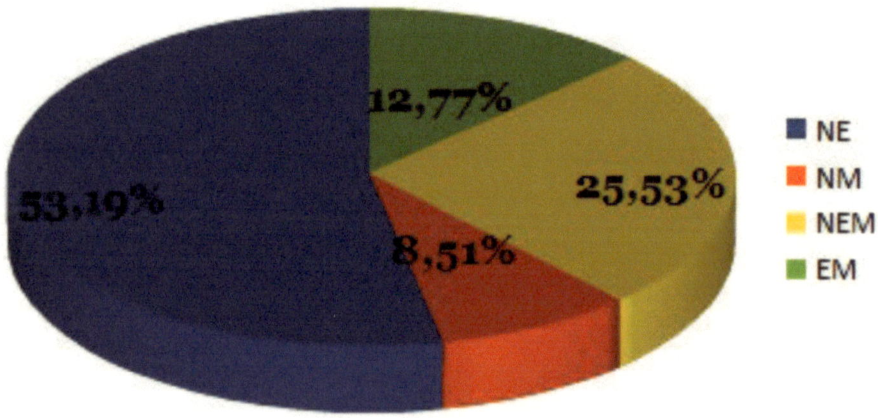

Figure 6.
Types of cells in mixed rhinosinusitis.

The picture that emerged from this evaluation allowed us to distinguish nasal pathologies in a practical and clear way on the basis of cytological aspects and therefore, in our opinion, to simplify their classification. Furthermore, the cytological characterization allows us to address the therapy in a very personal way and, in addition, to periodically evaluate the results in a more rigorous way.

We therefore distinguished the nasosinusal pathologies in groups based on the inflammatory cytotype most significantly represented in the analyzed sample:

- Neutrophilic rhinosinusitis
- Eosinophilic rhinosinusitis
- Mast cell rhinosinusitis

However, in some patients we found that it was not possible to define a dominant cytotype as the nasal mucosa was quantitatively similarly affected by more than one cell type. In these cases we use the term rhinosinusitis with mixed cellularity.

We then divided the mixed cellular rhinosinusitis into four subclasses:

- Neutrophilic-eosinophilic form
- Neutrophilic-mast cell form
- Neutrophil-eosinophil-mastocitary form
- Eosinophilic-mast cell form

3.1 Neutrophil rhinosinusitis

In our experience, it represents the most frequently encountered pathology. This condition is characterized by the more or less significant presence of inflammatory cells called neutrophils granulocytes.

The neutrophil granulocyte has a roundish shape and presents a clear ("neutral") cytoplasm with a purplish-red polylobate nucleus after MGG staining. The neutrophil granulocytes are distinguished in six different types based on the shape of the nucleus [2]. It is possible that the number of lobes is related to the age of the cell. In fact, in young granulocytes the nucleus often appears to be reniform, while in the older ones, it has different lobes.

The neutrophilic granulocyte plays an important immune function defending us from pathogenic microorganisms [6] and other irritating substances toward which it has an effective phagocytic activity. Once the phagocytosis process has been performed, a "killing" function is performed against pathogens thanks to the intracytoplasmic release of substances with a lithic action including hydrogen peroxide, superoxide ion, and some enzymes as elastase, lysozyme, collagenase, phosphatase, and lactoferrin.

According to Gelardi et al., the presence of sporadic neutrophils in the nasal mucosa would not represent an index of pathology. Instead, we have to make a diagnosis in case of high number of neutrophils. With infectious rhinosinusitis, the number of neutrophil granulocytes increases significantly. They are called back in the nasal mucosa in order to engulf the pathogenic microorganisms and eliminate them [7]. We observe in **Figure 7** some granulocytes with intracytoplasmic bacteria. In this image the moment immediately following the phagocytosis is shown, before the lithic enzymes are activated for digestive purposes. In the proposed image, we observe a bacterial infectious pathology. Microscopic observation can help us to differentiate the various types of germs involved in infection. We can in fact recognize the round shape of the bacteria as the *Staphylococcus Au*, the *Streptococcus Pn*, and the *Moraxella C.* or the elongated shape of the haemophilus I and the diphtheroids. Neutrophilic rhinosinusopathy with an infectious etiology may also present a viral or fungal etiology. In the latter case, we will observe the presence of fungal spores that present themselves with a particular "bulb" shape.

In infectious neutrophil rhinosinusitis, in addition to the increase in neutrophils and the presence of microbial agents (**Figure 8**), we will also be able to see an increase in lymphocytes, macrophages, and plasma cells and an increase in mucipar cells associated with decreased ciliated cells.

We found very interesting the observation of bluish areas that we define "infectious spots" [2]. Those represent the expression of bacterial biofilm or an exopolysaccharide matrix within which fungal bacteria and spores live. The structure of the biofilm would correspond to a sort of shell that guarantees pathogens a greater resistance to drugs.

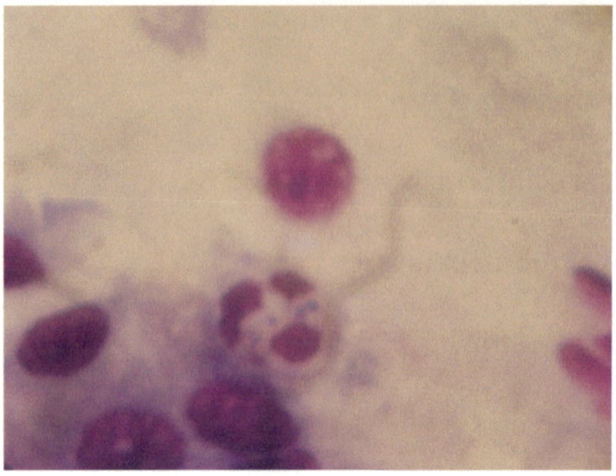

Figure 7.
Phagocytosis (neutrophil granulocyte with intracytoplasmic bacteria).

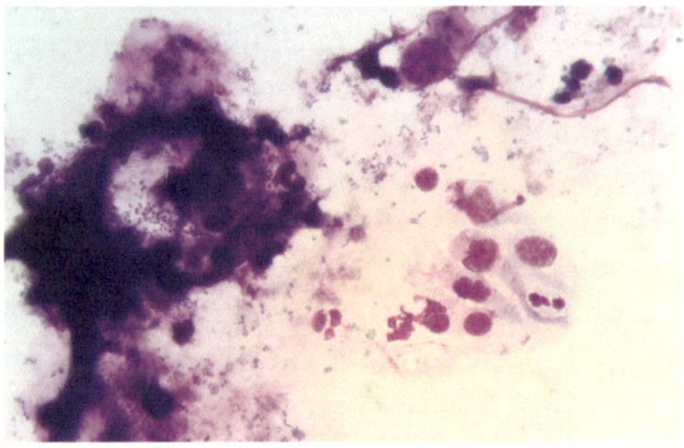

Figure 8.
Infectious neutrophil rhinosinusitis.

In the forms of viral etiology, we will not be able to find pathogenic microorganisms due to the insufficient magnification power of the optical microscope. However, we can observe some indirect signs of ciliated cells strongly suggestive of viral infection. In fact, they can present both alterations of the nuclear structure (polynucleation) and of the cytoplasmic component (inclusions and separations). Also usually in the viral infection, we observe an important increase of the lymphocytes. The finding of neutrophils in the nasal mucosa, however, also occurs in cases of noninfectious diseases. In these cases we can observe a variable number of neutrophil granulocytes without the cytological aspects described above. In this case, we are talking about a form of irritating rhinosinusitis in which often the etiologic agent is represented by a substance with an irritating action, which can be exogenous (powders, environmental pollutants, tobacco smoke, and toxic substances present in the professional field) or endogenous (gastroesophageal reflux disease) (**Figure 9**) [8].

In addition to the already described presence of neutrophils we can observe an alteration of the normal relationship between ciliate cells and muciparous cells. In fact, we often observe a reduction of the former and an increase in the latter. In other cases we can observe areas of squamous epithelium. According to some authors the severity of these rhinopathies would be associated with the number of neutrophils present.

In fact, by releasing their lithic enzymes and their toxic substances, they would cause damage to the respiratory mucosa proportional to the quantity of substances released.

Furthermore, in these patients, chronic mucosal damage and consequent alteration of mucociliary clearness would favor greater nasal fragility and a greater risk of contracting respiratory infections.

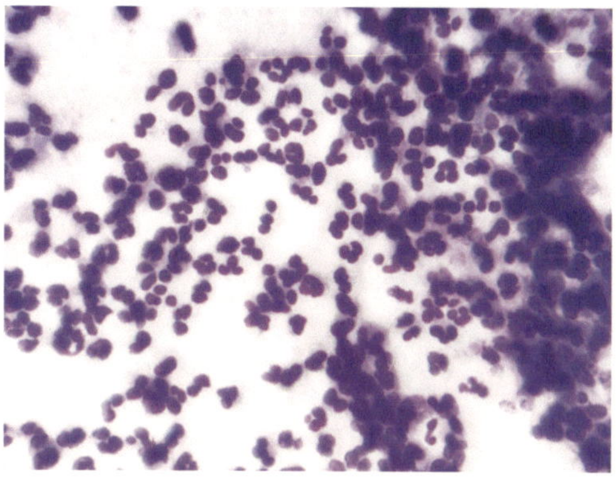

Figure 9.
Noninfectious neutrophil rhinosinusitis.

3.2 Eosinophilic rhinosinusitis

This condition is represented by the presence in the nasal mucosa of eosinophilic granulocytes. The eosinophilic granulocyte belongs, as well as neutrophil, to the group of leukocytes and also presents a roundish form, although of slightly greater dimensions. Frequently the nucleus appears bilobed (**Figure 10**).

The cytoplasm is of variable color from orange to intense pink, very distinctive and unmistakable. Inside, small granules are observed that contain substances such as the major basic protein (MBP), the eosinophilic cationic protein, and the eosinophilic peroxidase [9]. These substances have a cytotoxic and antibacterial function. In the cytoplasm of eosinophils, we also find enzymes (collagenase, phosphatase, and phospholipase) and substances derived from the metabolism of arachidonic acid as leukotrienes and prostaglandins (LTC4, PGD2, PGE1). These substances play a fundamental role in the mechanisms of inflammation, especially in the delayed phase of the allergic reaction (**Figure 11**).

The LTC4 leukotriene in particular has a bronchoconstriction action as well as prostaglandin PGD2, while prostaglandin E1 has a vasodilatory action. Other substances present in nongranular form in the cytoplasm of eosinophils are released

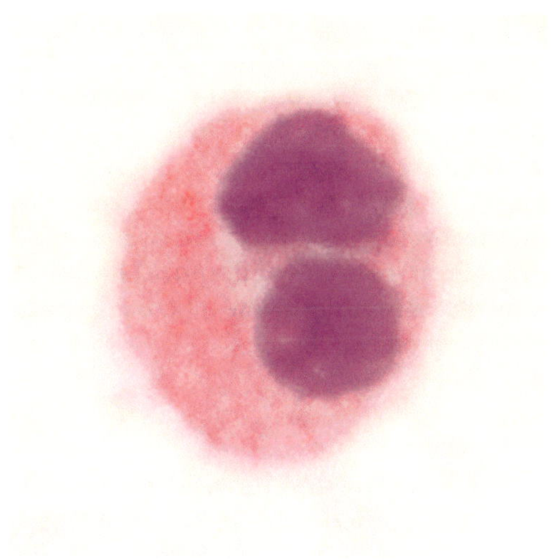

Figure 10.
Eosinophilous (frequently the nucleus appears bilobed).

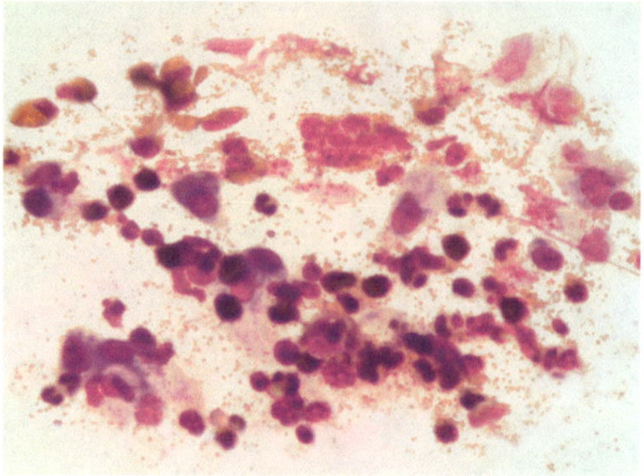

Figure 11.
Eosinophil rhinosinusitis (we observed an important degranulation reaction).

for chemotactic and amplification of the inflammatory processes. We recall among these IL2, which performs chemotactic action toward mast cells, IL3 with chemotactic action toward eosinophils, and IL5 with chemotactic action toward neutrophils [10].

Frequently we have found eosinophilic rhinosinusitis. Of 34 patients with this type of pathology, 38.24% (or 13 patients) had allergic rhinitis, the remainder suffered from other forms of rhinitis.

We have found in the 32.35% of subjects (11 patients) a vasomotoria rhinitis and in the 29.41% (10 patients) a nasal polyposis.

Eosinophilic rhinosinusitis has very specific clinical features. Affected patients complain of a very troublesome symptomatology, often characterized by sneezing and rhinorrhea, nasal itching, and nasal congestion. Symptoms can be triggered suddenly by the contact of the nasal mucosa with a known allergen, but also by the occurrence of some particular stimuli (such as sudden changes in temperature or humidity, contact with intense perfumes, tobacco smoke).

Patients with eosinophilic rhinosinusitis are often affected by other eosinophilic phenotype disorders such as bronchial asthma. For a long time, we have known that the course of the nasal pathology has a singular influence on the prognosis of the associated bronchial pathology. For this reason, a correct treatment and a good control of the nasal pathology are to be considered necessary.

We know that some granular components of eosinophils, such as major basic protein (MBP), have the ability to attack the desmosomal junctions by weakening the barrier action of the respiratory mucosa and exposing it to the action harmful to infectious chemical or physical agents [11]. Therefore patients suffering from eosinophilic rhinosinusitis not only suffer from symptoms that we could define direct and that are related to the action of components such as prostaglandins and leukotrienes but also indirect symptoms (purulent rhinorrhea, headache, pharyngodynia, cough, recurrent fever, episodes of dyspnea) derived from the overlap of other diseases favored by the weakening of the mucosal barrier and by the inefficiency of mucociliary clearance.

3.3 Mast cell rhinosinusitis

This condition is characterized by the presence of mast cells in the nasal mucosa. The mast cell is presented to the observation with a variable optical microscope: it can be vaguely roundish or lozenge shaped. It is characterized by a marked basophilia and has a coarsely oval nucleus generally covered by numerous granules (**Figure 12**). They are generally larger in size than eosinophilic granules.

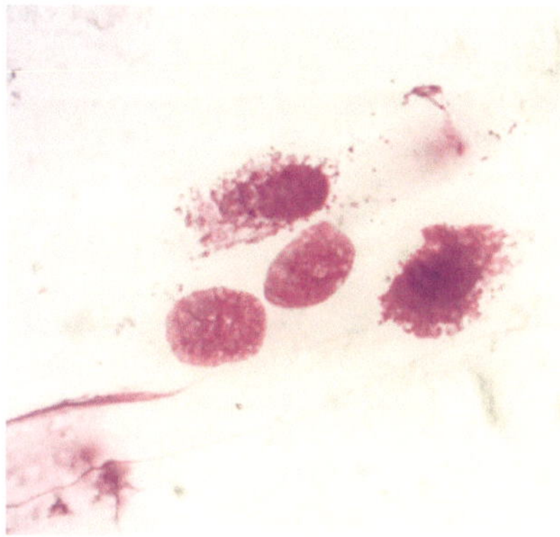

Figure 12.
Mast cell with degranulation.

The surface of mast cells is characterized by the presence of IgE receptors. When they bind to these receptors, the mast cell releases by exocytosis its granules with the substances contained therein including histamine, a preformed substance with multiple actions [12].

In fact, it acts on the vascular receptors favoring vasodilation and edema of the surrounding tissues. It also acts on the nasal glands, feeding the rhinorrhea, and stimulates the nerve endings favoring itching and sneezing. The mast cell through its granules also eliminates some preformed chemotactic factors such as IL4, IL5, and IL13. Arachidonic acid is also synthesized by newly formed metabolites such as PGD2 and LTC4, whose actions on smooth muscles and vessels have already been described previously.

The mast cell, once stimulated, determines immediate symptoms. This rapidity of action can be observed in the early phase of the allergic reaction [13]. However, this cell is able, through the release of chemotactic factors, to influence also late phlogistic reactions.

As we can show in **Figure 1**, mast cells are rarely the only cells involved in the pathogenesis of a rhinopathy. In fact, we found only 5 cases of mastocytic rhinosinusitis in 300 patients studied (1.67%). Of these patients two presented an allergic disease, while three patients had a nonallergic disease.

On the other hand, cases of mixed cellular pathologies with the presence of mast cells are very frequent.

Mast cell rhinosinusitis are characterized by very intense symptoms, characterized by marked nasal obstruction, serous rhinorrhoea, nasal pruritus, and sneezing. Also in this case as in eosinophilous cellularity diseases, we have reestablished an association with other pathologies with a similar phenotype such as bronchial asthma.

3.4 Mixed rhinosinusitis

We found a mixed rhinosinusitis in 94 patients corresponding to 32.75% of patients with rhinosinusitis and inflammatory phenotype (**Figure 1**). As we can see from the graph below, mixed rhinosinusitis is characterized by the presence in the nasal mucosa of several inflammatory cytotypes (**Figures 13** and **14**).

In 53.19% of the cases (50 patients), we found a pathology characterized by neutrophil and eosinophilic infiltration; in 25.53% of cases (24 patients), a type with neutrophilia-eosinophilia-mast cell; in 12.77% of cases (12 patients), eosinophilic and mast cell type and in 8; and 51% of the cases (8 patients), we found neutrophils and mast cells in the nasal mucosa. In many cases, mixed rhinosinusitis is found in

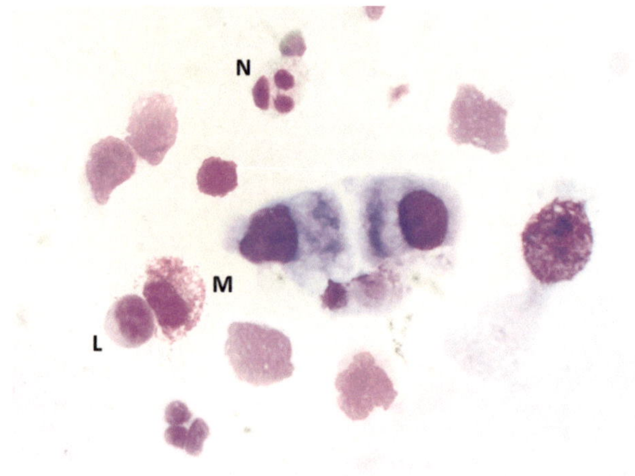

Figure 13.
Mixed rhinosinusitis with neutrophil (N), mast cell (M), and lymphocyte (L).

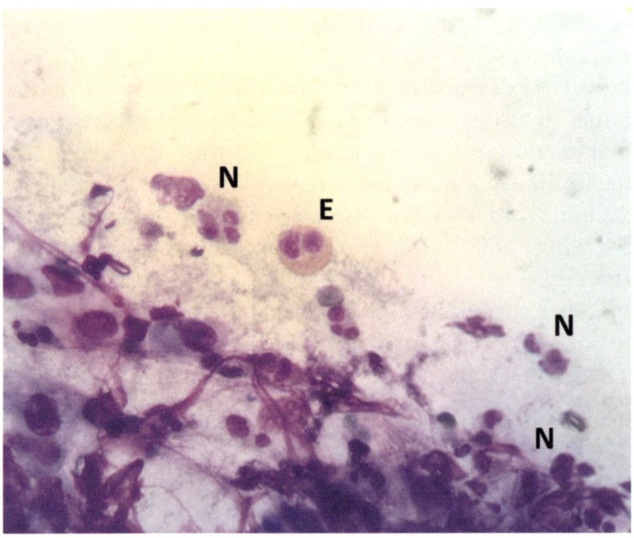

Figure 14.
Mixed rhinosinusitis with neutrophil (N) and eosinophil (E).

allergic patients. We have observed that a low intensity but stable and protracted allergenic stimulation, as in the case of allergies to Dermatophagoides, produces at a cytological level a framework defined by Gelardi et al. "Minimal persistent inflammation" is characterized by the presence of numerous neutrophil granulocytes and a small number of eosinophils or mast cells. Another interesting aspec is the greater association of the mixed forms with nasal polyposis compared to the other forms of rhinosinusitis as shown in the graph below (**Figures 15** and **16**).

We have indeed observed that in the category of rhinosinusitis with mixed cellularity, 23.40% of patients had developed a nasal polyposis, while in the other forms of rhinosinusitis, the percentage of patients who developed a nasal polyposis is lower (14.51%). The symptoms of this kind of disease varies according to the most characterizing cytotype. In any case we must remember how these forms are particularly harmful for the nasal mucosa and for mucociliary function, as they, according to our clinical experience, contribute in favoring an increased risk of respiratory inflammation in those affected.

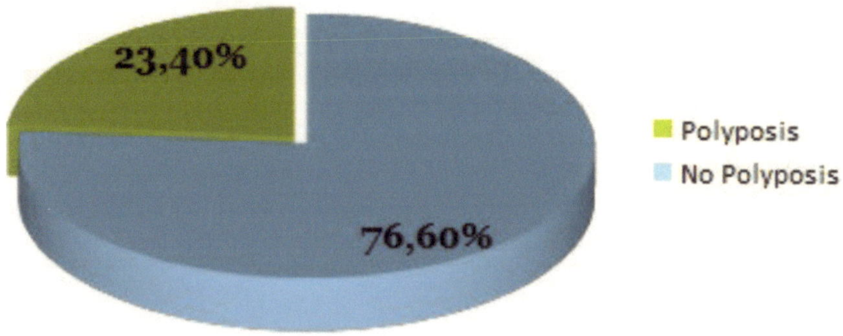

Figure 15.
Prevalence of polyposis in mixed rhinosinusitis.

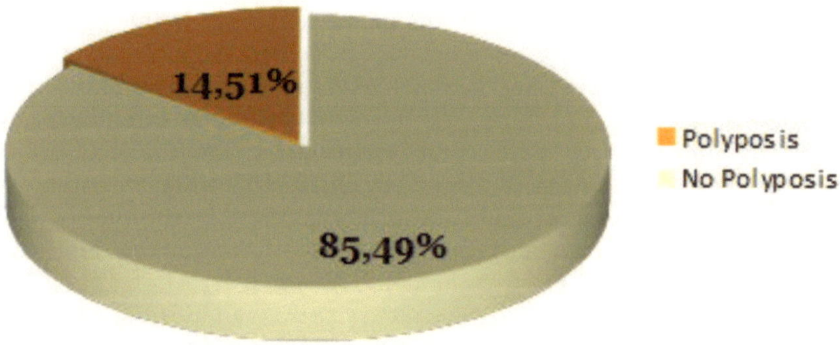

Figure 16.
Prevalence of polyposis in other types of rhinosinusitis.

4. Discussion

Our experience has allowed us to consider the nasal cytological examination as indispensable diagnostic tools for a better understanding of chronic inflammatory diseases of the rhinosinusal district.

Thanks to the information provided by the cytological examination, we can define the etiopathogenetic characteristics of the disease. Obviously the collection of the anamnesis represents a complementary and indispensable diagnostic element.

By carrying out these three diagnostic aspects, we are able to trace the identification of the pathology very precisely.

Daily experience has led us to acknowledge the necessity of a simplification regarding the classification of rhinosinusal diseases.

Once there was a clear demarcation between pathological processes at nasal localization, the rhinitis, from those with sinus localization, the sinusitis.

In agreement with the European guidelines present in the EPOS12 [14], we argue that very often the two pathologies are closely related, so that a clear border between the two is impossible. We therefore think it is practical as well as appropriate to use in clinical practice a single term that includes the two old forms of nasosinusal pathology. For these reasons, we will talk about chronic rhinosinusitis about any chronic inflammatory process that affects the rhinosinusal district.

The teaching of the pulmonologists, as explained in the GINA guidelines, led us to consider the nasal pathology narrow related to the bronchial situation. This is the reason why the phenotypic classification adopted for asthma is, in our opinion, extremely suitable also for the rhinosinusal pathology.

We have therefore redesigned the pneumological experience in order to use in our daily practice a simple and immediate distinction for the various forms of chronic rhinosinusitis. We have distinguished 2 large groups of pathologies based on the phenotype:

- Cellular rhinosinusites

- Noncellular rhinosinusitis

This first distinction in the 2 phenotypic classes arises from the firm belief that the clinical characteristics of the sinonasal pathology are closely related to the type of cell involved in the inflammatory process.

As shown in **Table 1**, in the cellular rhinosinusitis group, we contemplate the neutrophilic, eosinophilous, mast cell, and mixed cell forms. In the second group, (noncellular rhinosinusitis) we contemplate pathologies characterized by a normal cytological expression but equally characterized by sinonasal symptoms. Among these we include the iatrogenic forms, the hormonal forms, the atrophic forms, the mechanical forms (associated with septal dysmorphism), and the decubitus forms (characterized by significant nasal respiratory obstruction when the patient lies supine). In our case series, the number of patients affected by this type of pathology was much lower than patients affected by cellular rhinosinusitis. Precisely the individuals affected was 13 (equal to about 4.5%).

Indeed, the number of negative rhinocitograms was superior, almost three times as high. However, we have also included in the cellular group patients with negative cytological examination; in those cases we knew that the negative result originated from temporal circumstances. This applies, for example, to certain diseases with seasonal or recurring cellular characterizations. We have therefore attributed to the group of eosinophilic rhinosinusitis also those patients with clearly allergic symptoms and in which sensitization to seasonal allergens was ascertained despite having found in them a normal rhinocytogram. This situation occurs when we performed the sampling outside the allergy period.

We are sure of the central role of the cytotype in the sinonasal pathology manifestation, and we have also distinguished the mixed rhinosinusitis in four subclasses: the neutrophil-eosinophilic cellular form, the neutrophil-mast cell form, the neutrophil-eosinophil-mast cell form, and the eosinophilic-mast cell form.

This classification, with the support of an adequate imaging and with a correct anamnestic study, allows clinicians to diagnose all types of rhinosinusitis by means of an easy and intuitive classification.

The diagnostic classification performed by cytological examination allows a targeted therapeutic planning. In fact, the knowledge of the etiopathogenetic and cytological principles of a pathology allows a "tailor made" therapeutic planning and also allows to achieve a precise monitoring of the pathology. This leads to optimal control of symptoms and an inevitable prognostic improvement of chronic inflammatory diseases.

5. Conclusion

The classification of rhinosinusitis is still very complex and diversified today. Thanks to the information we can obtain from the nasal cytology and the anamnesis, we are able to easily frame the majority of rhinosinus pathologies in order to obtain a targeted therapeutic planning and adequate monitoring.

We have listed the pathologies observed and classified from the cytological point of view in 5 years of experience, and we have come to propose a simple and versatile classification that takes into account the different clinical and etiopathogenetic characteristics of the pathologies observed.

Based on the phenotype, we distinguished cellular rhinosinusitis from noncellular rhinosinusitis. The former are divided into four classes (the neutrophil form, the eosinophilic form, the mast cell form, and the mixed form). These types of rhinosinusitis are characterized by a specific cytological framework. We then grouped rhinosinusitis with a negative rhinocytogram in the noncellular phenotype. Among these we remember the iatrogenic forms, the forms on a hormonal base, the positional and decubitus, the atrophic, and the mechanical forms.

According to us, the distinction we have proposed is simple and immediate.

Acknowledgements

The author would like to thank Mauro Corinti for his contribution in photographic materials.

Conflict of interest

The author declares that there is no conflict of interest regarding the publication of this paper.

Notes/thanks/other declarations

Thanks to Giorgia Bottani for general support and assistance.

Author details

Marco Capelli
Columbus Clinic Center, Milan, Italy

*Address all correspondence to: info@otorinocremona.it

References

[1] Galarza-Paez L, Anatomy DBW. Treasure Island. FL: StatPearls Publishing; 2018. p. 22

[2] Gelardi M. Atlante di citologia nasale—per la diagnosi differenziale delle rinopatie. 2nd ed. Milano: Ermes SRL; 2012

[3] Piqué N, De Servi B. Rhinosectan® spray (containing xyloglucan) on the ciliary function of the nasal respiratory epithelium; results of an in vitro study. Allergy, Asthma and Clinical Immunology. 2018;**14**:41. DOI: 10.1186/s13223-018-0268-3

[4] Rouadi P, Baroody FM, Abbott D, Naureckas E, Solway J, Naclerio RM. A technique to measure the ability of the human nose to warm and humidify air. Journal of Applied Physiology. 1999;**87**(1):400-406

[5] Freeman SC, Kahwaji CI. Treasure Island. FL: StatPearls Publishing; 2018. p. 27

[6] Hergott CB, Roche AM, Naidu NA, Mesaros C, Blair IA. Weiser bacterial exploitation of phosphorylcholine mimicry suppresses inflammation to promote airway infection. The Journal of Clinical Investigation. 2015;**125**(10):3878-3890. DOI: 10.1172/JCI81888

[7] Kolaczkowska E, Kubes P. Neutrophil recruitment and function in health and inflammation. Nature Reviews. Immunology. 2013;**13**(3):159-175. DOI: 10.1038/nri3399

[8] Caruso AA, Del Prete S, Ferrara L, Serra R, Telesca DA, Ruggiero S, et al. Relationship between gastroesophageal reflux disease and Ph nose and salivary: Proposal of a simple method outpatient in patients adults. Open Medicine. 2016;**11**(1):381-386. DOI: 10.1515/med-2016-0069

[9] Zhu X, Liu K, Wang J, Peng H, Pan Q, Wu S, et al. C-C chemokine receptor type 3 gene knockout alleviates inflammatory responses in allergic rhinitis model mice by regulating the expression of eosinophil granule proteins and immune factors. Molecular Medicine Reports. 2018;**18**(4):3780-3790. DOI: 10.3892/mmr.2018.9380

[10] Varricchi G, Bagnasco D, Borriello F, Heffler E, Canonica GW. Interleukin-5 pathway inhibition in the treatment of eosinophilic respiratory disorders: Evidence and unmet needs. Current Opinion in Allergy and Clinical Immunology. 2016;**16**(2):186-200

[11] Acharya KR, Hogan SP. Eosinophil granule proteins: Form and function. The Journal of Biological Chemistry. 2014;**289**(25):17406-17415

[12] Vukman KV, Försönits A, Oszvald Á, Tóth E, Buzás E. Mast cell secretome: Soluble and vesicular components. Seminars in Cell & Developmental Biology. 2017;**67**:65-73

[13] Korošec P, Gibbs BF, Rijavec M, Custovic A, Turner PJ. Important and specific role for basophils in acute allergic reactions. Clinical and Experimental Allergy. 2018;**48**(5):502-512

[14] Fokkens WJ, Lund VJ, Mullol J, Bachert C, Alobid I, Baroody F, et al. EPOS 2012: European position paper on rhinosinusitis and nasal polyps 2012. A summary for otorhinolaryngologists. Rhinology. 2012;**50**(1):1-12

Chapter 4

Chronic Sinusitis: The Empiric Treatment Strikes Back: Is CRS Directly Caused by Infectious Agent(s)?

Alexander Nowicki, Natalie Nowicki, Stella Nowicki, Alfred Samet, Michal Michalik, Roger Su, James K. Fortson and Bogdan Nowicki

Abstract

Chronic sinusitis leads to unresolved infection and inflammation resulting in tissue remodeling, then further propagates the vicious cycle of deterioration and dysfunction of the sinuses' natural defense mechanisms, and yet another cycle of infection and mucosal injury. Antibiotic therapy targeting pathogens classically implicated in sinusitis could augment the risk of therapeutic failure through the natural selection of resistant and/or virulent pathogens, especially in the presence of Gram-negative *E. coli*. Our recent demonstration of highly pathogenic *E. coli,* detected through intraoperative biopsy of sinus tissue, allowed the resolution of chronic sinusitis symptoms upon *E. coli* targeted therapy. The isolated *E. coli* carried three genes, each coding biofilm formation, which may, in part, account for the chronicity of *E. coli* sinusitis. We recommend that, patients with chronic sinusitis be considered for intraoperative biopsy for unusual pathogens, therefore allowing targeted therapy. In the future, use of vaccines and biofilm inhibitors might be an effective therapeutic consideration.

Keywords: chronic sinusitis, rhinosinusitis, *E. coli*, biofilm, genotype, virulence factors, antibiotic treatment, antibiotic resistance, biopsy

1. Introduction

1.1 Is CRS directly caused by infectious agents?

Our current state of knowledge indicates that chronic rhinosinusitis (CRS) is not directly caused by infectious agents [1]. Instead, the current paradigm states that CRS is a spectrum of "self-perpetuating" non-infectious inflammatory processes. If this is the case, that would mean that repetitive, long term, systemic antibiotic therapy has little to no role in the treatment of CRS, except in the event of an acute exacerbation. Furthermore, this would suggest that clinical improvement of CRS would be more appropriately explained by the reduction of inflammatory injury as a whole, and only secondarily by the amelioration of bacterial load and the resultant removal of super-antigens.

Albeit this working theory pivots upon a non-infectious etiology it does raise many concerns in the direction of microbiology. The most paramount of which is that the misappropriate, frequent, and long term use of antibiotics actually selects for a pathological microflora, composed of microorganisms resistant to antibiotics, which may also form biofilms that may never be eradicated [1]. These biofilms may then act as the perfect stage for future acute exacerbations, functioning as a protective bunker for bacteria lying dormant within the film, and even create quasi-resistant bacteria. For example, a naturally antibiotic-sensitive bacterium contained within a biofilm may be out of reach of the action of an antibiotic, rendering it resistant-in-vivo.

This idea is closely paralleled and supported by animal models of *Pseudomonas*-biofilm formation within sinus mucosa; where, *Pseudomonas*-biofilm required 400 times the concentration of tobramycin to be eradicated. Similarly, topical antibiotics are frequently ineffective at standard doses, which is often considered clinical proof of the non-bacterial etiology of CRS [2]. However, whether or not the proposed explanations are clinically valid for a non-bacterial mechanism of CRS remains a debatable issue and should be carefully evaluated in the context of published studies.

Now, we will review these questions in a step-by-step fashion: physiology, sinus microflora, and recent discoveries on the role of punch biopsy in CRS and its detection of deep-tissue sinus infection.

2. Is a healthy sinus cavity free of bacteria?

So, now the question is, is sterility synonymous with well-being? By using microbiome technology to detect difficult to culture bacteria, it was observed that bacteria are present in both healthy and diseased sinuses [3]. However, a pilot study on CRS patients actually discovered a significantly lower taxa of bacteria than their healthy control. So, at first glance it may look like the opposite, a lower number of bacteria is correlated with a higher likelihood of CRS. Does this point to a non-infectious etiology, then?

Importantly, these microbiome studies did not only reveal a difference in absolute number of bacteria, but in the content of the bacterial flora. Further analysis revealed that the bacterial taxa of the CRS patients was largely defined by relatively high numbers of unique single species, such as *Corynebacterium tuberculostearicum*, while microbiome analysis in the healthy control group showed a relative abundance of *Lactobacillus* spp., *Enterococcus* spp., and *Pediococcus* spp., but what does all of this mean in practice? These findings suggest that the etiology of CRS may hinge upon balance and equilibrium, and not at all upon bacterial load.

To investigate this hypothesis further, a study was designed on a mouse model of inflammatory sinusitis. This study revealed something extremely interesting. Sinus infection by *C. tuberculostearicum* led to hyperplasia [3], but not by itself. This hyperplasia only occurred with the administration of antibiotics. It looks that the use of antibiotics backfired. Upon antibiotic treatment the commensal bacteria of the healthy sinus cavity were eliminated, selecting for an antibiotic resistant strain *C. tuberculostearicum,* which became opportunistically pathogenic without a commensal microflora to police its growth. But what would happen if we rebalanced our flora? Could this process be reversed?

Interestingly enough, upon the addition of the *Lactobacillus sakei* the process reversed entirely, returning the sinus cavity to its natural state. The conclusion of this intriguing study was that antibiotic treatment of acute rhinosinusitis may be a "Catch-22", and although it may rid the body of the archetypal bacteria of acute sinusitis, it may contribute to the future development of persistent sinusitis and/or CRS. These findings spark many questions and begin to steer the medical mind toward similar situations within different specialties.

Taking these discoveries of bacterial imbalance into consideration, it may be appropriate to draw analogies across specialties, and explore the realm of microbiotic imbalance in the upper respiratory tract as it relates to the female urogenital tract. We may be able to draw important conclusions in the pathogenesis of floral-imbalance-induced-CRS through the data analysis of microbiome studies in bacterial vaginosis (BV). BV is an infection in which anaerobic bacteria overgrow vaginal mucosa as a direct result of the, often inadvertent, elimination of Lactobacillus species [4]. These species naturally secret bactericidal H_2O_2 that kills anaerobic species—protecting the delicate membranes of the vaginal mucosa. Just as CRS, BV is frequently a recurrent process. However, a very simple single treatment with Metronidazole and/or recolonization with Lactobacillus often restores the health of mucosal membranes. It may be an oversimplification of a complex disease state, but the possibility of a similar etiology and therefore similar non-invasive cost-effective treatment is tantalizing.

2.1 Alternative thesis: CRS involves direct bacterial infection

As much evidence as there may be for the noninfectious hypothesis of CRS, there is just as much supporting the opposite. So where does the truth lie? As with most things in life, most likely somewhere in the middle. Either way, here we will explore the possibility of infectious CRS, and some of the most recent discoveries and theories behind it.

The noninfectious hypothesis of CRS is certainly a tantalizing one, but it is strongly challenged by the alternative hypothesis [5]. The authors of this chapter tend to lean toward the more active process of infection as the most common etiology, and we propose that the predominant progression of CRS directly involves bacterial infection. Furthermore, we believe that most of the theories and concepts pointing toward a noninfectious etiology, have been improperly evaluated and interpreted, and when reanalyzed tend to support an infectious cause of CRS.

Many parallels can be drawn between the two main arguments, one of which is the selection of microflora and or pathogens by inadequate or improper antimicrobial treatment. Some pathogens, such as *E. coli*, are able to both actively and passively elude destruction and clearance through multiple mechanisms, and current studies are pointing toward the fact that we as clinicians are inadvertently selecting for them. Through mechanisms similar to those described in the previous sections, incomplete treatment of bacterial sinusitis looks to be inducing the escape of such organisms from the reach of the immune system as a whole, as well as antibiotics specifically, by driving these microorganisms into our body's white cells or deep within the sinus mucosa. Simultaneously, the resultant disruption of the commensal bacterial community and mucosal integrity of the sinus leads to the formation of biofilm, which in our opinion is both a strong supplementary contributor and a direct cause of subacute and chronic infectious processes.

As discussed previously, a weakened microflora may contribute to the dysfunction of the sinus mucosa and disruption of the general local immune state. This, in combination with a slew of other complex factors, creates the perfect platform for the formation of a biofilm. Once formed, biofilm contributes to the failure of the antibiotic treatment by preventing any significant antibiotic penetration. Bacteria hiding within the structure of the film, become effectively invulnerable, when in any other situation they would be easily eliminated. As an added layer to the issue, superficial swab and culture of the mucosal surface may be completely misleading.

A positive bacterial culture of the biofilm showing in vitro antibiotic sensitivity may misdirect therapy entirely. Although you've confirmed in vitro effectiveness of therapy in regard to your surface culture, the chosen antimicrobial will most likely miss any pathogen lying deep within the film, interstitium, or intracellular space, rendering the chosen treatment clinically moot when used in-vivo.

Now put yourself in the shoes of the clinician. You've swabbed properly and sent for culture and sensitivity, then treated accordingly, but there is no clinical improvement in your patient's state of health. So, what do you do next? What conclusions may you draw? Such a cycle of negligible response to antibiotic therapy may inappropriately perpetuate the idea of pathogen independent CRS, when in reality it should raise questions of drug choice, administration, and adjunct therapy.

This thought process brings one particular example to mind and into question. Recently Antunes et al. showed that a *Pseudomonas* containing biofilm required 400 times the concentration of tobramycin to be eradicated than its control counterpart. While this finding became a warning, heeded by many, against the "ineffective" antibiotic treatment of biofilm, and even further, considered by some as the disproval of a bacterial origin of CRS, this may be a grave misunderstanding. Looking back to our foundations in pharmacology we must remember that many antibiotics have near-no activity on intracellular pathogens hiding within white or epithelial cells [6]. A fantastic real-world example of this being the aminoglycosides, like tobramycin, in particular.

In the world of microbiology the classic model for establishing intracellular infection in vitro is achieved by introducing an aminoglycoside to the infected epithelial cell culture. Once introduced the aminoglycoside does in fact eliminate the extracellular bacteria, however counterintuitively it actually positively selects for the intracellular pathogens. This pharmacological model is well established in many fields of microbiology and Infectious Disease research, often exploited in many classic experimental algorithms, across many specialties—except, it seems, for those in the area of ENT and CRS [6]. Such an oversight may have immensely detrimental effects on the validity of conclusions drawn from an otherwise extremely important finding.

The current paradigm of thought, that chronic rhinosinusitis has no direct infectious etiology, is further challenged by the clinical efficacy of treatment with Mupirocin lavage in CRS patients who had positive endoscopically guided cultures for *Staphylococcus aureus* [7]. In one recent investigation of CRS, 15 of 16 patients treated with Mupirocin-saline nasal irrigation, twice daily for 3 weeks, saw significant clinical improvement followed by a negative repeat culture for *S. aureus after* treatment. A follow-up double-blinded, placebo-controlled, study on 22 patients with CRS non-responsive to surgery demonstrated infection clearance in 8 of 9 patients after 1 month of mupirocin treatment [8]. Although the clinical improvement could be explained by the resolution of an acute exacerbation or the elimination of *Staphylococcus* super-antigens, these studies clearly challenge the current dogma of noninfectious CRS, and furthermore may directly support a pathogenic etiology of chronic sinusitis.

3. Finding *E. coli* in patients chronically ill with sinusitis

There is much left to understand and discover about the pathogenesis of CRS, from both the infectious and non-infectious standpoints, and it will be many years before we have a full grasp on the matter, if ever. In the meantime, many groups are publishing some interesting studies with very exciting results, and conclusions.

Recently, we have reported on the importance of proper biopsy in chronic sinusitis, and how such data may influence treatment and outcomes [5]. Interestingly, the predominance of specific pathogens differs in congruence with the method of sample collection. For instance, with swab and culture bacterial growth is most commonly dominated by the classic Gram-positives implicated in sinusitis. However, when samples are collected intraoperatively, by punch biopsy, the script is flipped and a predominance of Gram-negatives, including *E. coli*, is found [9, 10]. Therefore, logic dictates that if antibiotic therapy targets only the classic culprits of sinusitis, with Gram-negatives present, we may be achieving an incomplete or even inappropriate eradication of microflora and pathogens. This could explain and contribute to therapeutic failure in recurrent sinusitis, its transition into chronicity, and its interpretation as noninfectious [11–19].

In general, the presence of nonclassical pathogens such as Gram-negatives, namely *E. coli*, has been poorly documented. However, more and more groups are finding *E. coli* in patients chronically ill with sinusitis, and the question remains, "Are these contaminants, or are they true pathogens?". By definition if the latter is true, and these isolated *E. coli* are pathogenic, there should be evidence of their ability to produce disease, through the demonstration of various virulence factors [20–22]. Alternatively, if they are non-pathogenic and represent random contamination or commensal properties then there should be no evidence of genetic markers of virulence. So far, the nature of *E. coli* virulence and potential for cause of CRS remains largely unknown [23–26]; and while numerous studies have explored the role of virulence genes in chronic and recurrent GI and Urinary Tract infections, no such data has been available in regard to chronic sinusitis, until recently [5, 23–25].

We recently published the first report demonstrating an association between a highly pathogenic *E. coli*, chronic sinusitis, and the resolution of symptoms upon *E. coli* targeted therapy [5]. Our findings support the theory that a non-classical pathogen may lurk below the radar in non-pharmacologically-responsive CRS and would only be detected by the use of proper techniques. When we performed intraoperative biopsy and culture on our chronic sinusitis patients, followed by genetic analysis of virulence factors, we found the presence of a clearly non-random pathogenic *E. coli*. These *E. coli* carried genes encoding multiple virulence factors, granting them the ability to produce biofilm. Upon catering our antibiotic therapy to each patient's biopsy and culture, we were able to obtain long term resolution of symptoms. These results, as a whole, lead us to believe that there very well may be genetic uniformity amongst *E. coli* isolated from patients suffering from CRS. These are not randomly occurring colonizers, or opportunistic colonizers.

3.1 Genetic analysis discover highly pathogenic *E. coli* in CRS

Generally, *E. coli* can be grouped genetically. Commonly, commensal *E. coli* are placed in phylogenetic groups A or B1, while pathogenic isolates are grouped in B2 or D [27, 28]. Upon in-depth genetic analysis of these patients, we found that 77% of isolated *E. coli* belonged to the pathogenic phylogenetic group B2, while only 23% belonged to the commensal B1 group [5]. This is concerning, not only due to shear pathogenicity, but the numerous dangerous traits associated with the bacteria in group B2. *E. coli* within this group are commonly capable of iron acquisition, granting them the ability to invade cells and multiply intracellularly and even within the blood stream. This makes members of the phylogenetic group B2 particularly toxic—contributing greatly to the inflammatory process and tissue injury of chronic infection.

Diving deeper, we find that these *E. coli* share many attributes with extraintestinal-pathogenic-*E. coli*. However, other features suggest that they might be specifically pathogenic to sinus tissue [29, 30]. One example of this tissue specificity is the *sfa* adhesin gene, normally associated with meningitis [31]. It is no stretch of the imagination to think that two anatomical structures, in such close proximity as the sinuses and the meninges, may be invaded through similar cytophysiological pathways. Especially by multiple bacteria with a generally enigmatic local affinity, whom happen to share virulence factors. This association needs to be explored further, but for now it is exciting to think that we may be able to better explain local affinity (tropism) to the head and neck through such mechanisms.

Other highlights of this genetic analysis include the finding of both the *hly*A and *usp* genes. These genes encode for the formation of bacterial toxins and are only present in highly virulent bacterial strains. In this patient group, they were present in over 70% of the *E. coli* isolates. By the other side of the same token, isolates were found to lack *dra*/*afa* adhesins, which are implicated in chronic and recurrent UTI and gestational pyelonephritis. Such a bold distinction may further support the idea that these isolates represent a novel subset of *E. coli*, with a unique genome, and possibly even tropism for the mucosa of the paranasal sinuses [32].

Unexpectedly, there were three genes that were found in 100% of isolated *E. coli* from our patients. These genes were agn43, fimG/H, and fyuA [33–36]. All of which are associated with UTI, and play a role in biofilm formation: agn43 assists in *E. coli*-*E. coli* self-adhesion, fimG/H codes for type 1 fimbriae allowing for *E. coli* to aggregate and adhere to mannose receptors on mucosal membranes, while fyuA assists in iron scavenging and is often implicated in septicemia.

Possibly most shocking of all is that, when analyzed via a pseudo-phylogenetic tree, these genes had closely associated genetic loci, which signifies a very probable cooperation amongst them. This raises a very concerning question. Could these three genes, working together, code for some sort of "super biofilm"? This could explain how and why so many mono-therapies and empiric treatments fail to yield any improvement in patients who suffer from CRS. A biofilm of this nature would in essence be both a defensive and offensive fortification for the pathogen. A sort of moated fortress with large watch towers, never allowing antibiotics or the host immune system to penetrate it, creating an ideal environment for lingering infection and chronic inflammation.

The resolution of CRS—following FESS, intra-operative biopsy, and antibiotic therapy targeted toward the resultant culture and sensitivity—is highly suggestive of *E. coli*'s strong contribution to the disease state of this patient population. Undoubtedly, this all hinges upon the genetic makeup of these bacteria, and the fact that their genetic code is set for pathogenesis by carrying the information necessary to express virulence factors, including the production of biofilm [37, 38]. Further deductive reasoning leads us to believe that, *E. coli* is a generally undermined and undetected etiologic factor of CRS and a major contributor of inflammation in these patients. Whether or not the presence of biofilm producing *E. coli* is directly responsible for the poor therapeutic response, after FESS alone, will continue to be explored in more detail [39–42].

As with all, there are limitations to this study that should be recognized. For example, the present investigation was a study of healthcare-seeking adults; only including those that were *E. coli* positive, raising a very important question. To what extent do these results apply to the general population? Next, due to the resolution of symptoms and subsequently negative cultures, along with consideration for cost and patient comfort, we did not perform a follow-up punch biopsy and analysis.

4. Future studies

Future studies should investigate the role of important factors in human health, such as the effects of hormones, like estrogen and progesterone, on chronic sinusitis [43, 44]. Which are known to control the immune system. We must also further explore the effects of obesity and diabetes mellitus on the risk of infection, as well as the relation of anatomical structure and function on the role of bacterial colonization. All of these factors change the expression of mucosal receptors, which is often exploited by various bacterial species, easing colonization and/or infection [32, 45].

In regard to the possibility of hormonal control of the immune system of the upper respiratory tract, we speculate that the head and neck may be analogous to the female urogenital tract. Wherein sensitivity to infection rises during the secretory and proliferative phases of the menstrual cycle [44]. Exploring further in this direction, the anatomical structure of the upper respiratory system appears to resemble the urogenital tract in many ways. Within the urinary tract an ascending infection begins with the colonization of vaginal introitus, before migrating proximally [21]. Genital colonization with *E. coli* may progress to infection of the urethra, which then ascends to the bladder, and further up to the kidneys via the ureters. This is made possible through the exploitation of tissue specific receptors to which bacteria anchor via specialized adherence structures called fimbriae [46, 47]. This process of bacterial migration results in acute pyelonephritis, often followed by chronic kidney infection with even further spread to the blood stream and resultant urosepticemia [48–50]. Similarly, we implore the medical community to consider the oropharynx, nasal cavities and paranasal sinuses as another anatomical system conducive to similar ascending infections [21, 45]. Beginning with the colonization of the oral and nasal cavities, bacteria may migrate "upstream" to the maxillary and then frontal sinuses, as well as others along the way via similar receptor-ligand interaction. All of which may be complicated by anatomical variation, anomaly, and pathology, ranging from nasal polyps and turbinate hypertrophy to choanal atresia and structural issues of the sort. These problems may be caused by everything from allergy to genetic mutation—resulting in a slew of aggravating factors, expression of specialized epithelial cell types, and tissue receptors—all contributing to the risk of chronic rhinosinusitis.

5. Considerations and conclusions

All things considered, chronic sinusitis remains a bit of an enigma. However, the more we explore the better we will be able to understand the complex multifactorial etiology that's sure to be lying below the surface. That being said, we've learned and discovered so much as a medical community in recent years, we believe there is no better time than now to begin making the most of it.

Keeping in mind the most recent publications and studies, we urge physicians to consider intraoperative punch biopsy on all of their chronic sinusitis patients [5]. Biopsied samples should be homogenized, and host cells should be exposed to membrane destabilizing buffers, lysing them and releasing trapped intracellular bacteria, allowing for the most thorough culture and analysis. Considering that a direct culture of the sample on solid media may not always be fruitful, we recommend the use of liquid media which may better allow the growth and detection of bacteria, even at low numbers. Next, cultures should be tested individually for antibiotic sensitivity and a personalized therapy should be prescribed to each individual patient. Finally, we also urge you to consider sending bacterial isolates for genotyping [35, 48, 51–57]. Through doing so we can finally stop asking of ourselves if we're fighting the right bug and know for certain that if it expresses virulence it is part of the problem.

We believe that through the use of these methods we may be able to better differentiate between specific etiologies of CRS within our patients, and through doing so we hope that we can avoid inappropriate antibiotic use, repeat surgeries, and prolonged treatment. Giving our patients their health and quality of life back faster and more effectively than ever.

In conclusion, we hope that personalized medicine may one day overshadow empiric treatment in chronic sinusitis, and all of our patients will be catered to with the utmost efficiency. With further testing and experimentation, we may be able to someday use vaccines or bacterial adhesion blockers to augment our therapies [30, 58]. Using genotyping to pick and choose what's best for our patients, we may be able to target specific virulence factors that allow such abilities as iron binding or cellular adherence, effectively rendering those bacterial invaders non-pathogenic. Through interdisciplinary exploration we may be able to adopt and adapt what other specialties have learned and use it to restore mucosal and micro-floral balance, and band together to fight bacteria and biofilm together as a medical community.

Acknowledgements

We thank you Nowicki Institute for Women's Health Research, Nashville, Tennessee, USA for support.

Conflict of interest

Authors declare no conflict of interest.

Author details

Alexander Nowicki[1], Natalie Nowicki[1], Stella Nowicki[2], Alfred Samet[3], Michal Michalik[3], Roger Su[4], James K. Fortson[4] and Bogdan Nowicki[2]*

1 Washington University of Health and Science, Nowicki Institute for Women's Health Research, Nashville, Tennessee, USA

2 Nowicki Institute for Women's Health Research, Nashville, Tennessee, USA

3 Medical Center MML, Warsaw, Poland

4 ENT Associates of South Atlanta, East Point, GA, USA

*Address all correspondence to: bnowicki1949@gmail.com

References

[1] Kennedy JL, Borish L. Chronic rhinosinusitis and antibiotics: The good, the bad, and the ugly. The American Journal of Rhinology and Allergy. 2013;**27**(6):467-472. DOI: 10.2500/ajra.2013.27.3960

[2] Antunes MB, Feldman MD, Cohen NA, Chiu AG. Dose-dependent effects of topical tobramycin in an animal model of *Pseudomonas sinusitis*. American Journal of Rhinology. 2007;**21**:423-427

[3] Abreu NA, Nagalingam NA, Song Y, Roediger FC, Pletcher SD, Goldberg AN, et al. Sinus microbiome diversity depletion and *Corynebacterium tuberculostearicum* enrichment mediates rhinosinusitis. Science Translational Medicine. 2012;**4**:151ra124

[4] Ma B, Forney LJ, Ravel J. Vaginal microbiome: Rethinking health and disease. Annual Review of Microbiology. 2012;**66**:371-389. DOI: 10.1146/annurev-micro-092611-150157

[5] Michalik M, Samet A, Marszałek A, Krawczyk B, Kotłowski R, Nowicki A, et al. *Escherichia coli* that carry fimG/H, fyuA and agn43 genes coding biofilm formation. 2018;**13**(3):e0192899. DOI: 10.1371/journal.pone.0192899.e. Collection 2018

[6] Rana T, Hasan RJ, Nowicki S, Venkatarajan MS, Singh R, Urvil PT, et al. Complement protective epitopes and CD55-microtubule complexes facilitate the invasion and intracellular persistence of uropathogenic *Escherichia coli*. Journal of Infectious Diseases. 2014;**209**(7):1066-1076

[7] Uren B, Psaltis A, Wormald PJ. Nasal lavage with mupirocin for the treatment of surgically recalcitrant chronic rhinosinusitis. Laryngoscope. 2008;**118**:1677-1680

[8] Jervis-Bardy J, Boase S, Psaltis A, et al. A randomized trial of mupirocin sinonasal rinses versus saline in surgically recalcitrant staphylococcal chronic rhinosinusitis. Laryngoscope. 2012;**122**:2148-2153

[9] Stevens WW, Lee RJ, Schleimer RP, Cohen NA. Chronic rhinosinusitis pathogenesis. The Journal of Allergy and Clinical Immunology. 2015;**136**(6):1442-1453

[10] Udayasri B, Radhakumari T. Microbial etiology of chronic sinusitis. Journal in Dental Science and Medical Science. 2016;**15**(1):118-124

[11] Halawi AM, Smith SS, Chandra RK. Chronic rhinosinusitis: Epidemiology and cost. Allergy and Asthma Proceedings. 2013;**34**(4):328-334

[12] Ivanchenko OA, Karpishchenko SA, Kozlov RS, Krechikova OI, Otvagin IV, Sopko ON, et al. The microbiome of the maxillary sinus and middle nasal meatus in chronic rhinosinusitis. Rhinology. 2016;**54**(1):68-74

[13] Manes RP, Batra PS. Etiology, diagnosis and management of chronic rhinosinusitis. Expert Review of Anti-Infective Therapy. 2013;**11**(1):25-35

[14] Oakley GM, Curtin K, Orb Q, Schaefer C, Orlandi RR, Alt JA. Familial risk of chronic rhinosinusitis with and without nasal polyposis: Genetics or environment. International Forum of Allergy and Rhinologyis. 2015;**5**(4):276-282

[15] Soler ZM, Mace JC, Litvack JR, Smith TL. Chronic rhinosinusitis, race, and ethnicity. American Journal of Rhinology and Allergy. 2012;**26**(2):110-116

[16] Lam K, Schleimer R, Kern RC. The etiology and pathogenesis of chronic

rhinosinusitis: A review of current hypotheses. Current Allergy and Asthma Reports. 2015;**15**(7):41

[17] Stephenson MF, Mfuna L, Dowd SE. Molecular characterization of the polymicrobial flora in chronic rhinosinusitis. Journal of Otolaryngology–Head and Neck Surgery. 2010;**39**:182-187

[18] Stressmann FA, Rogers GB, Chan SW. Characterization of bacterial community diversity in chronic rhinosinusitis infections using novel culture-independent techniques. The American Journal of Rhinology and Allergy. 2011;**25**:e133e140

[19] Hamad WA, Matar N, Elias M. Bacterial flora in normal adult maxillary sinuses. American Journal of Rhinology and Allergy. 2009;**23**:261-263

[20] Nowicki B, Sledzinska A, Samet A, Nowicki S. Pathogenesis of gestational UTI: Urinary obstruction vs. immune adaptation and microbial virulence. BJOG: An International Journal of Obstetrics and Gynaecology. 2011;**118**(2):109-112

[21] Nowicki B. In vitro models for the study of uropathogens. In: Mobley HLT, Warren JW, editors. Urinary Tract Infection: Molecular Pathogenesis to Clinical Management. Washington, DC: American Society for Microbiology; 1996. pp. 341-376

[22] Spaulding CN, Hultgren SJ. Adhesive pili in UTI pathogenesis and drug development. Pathogens. 2016;**5**(1):30. ASM Press. pp. 341-369

[23] Kremer B, Jacobs JA, Soudijn ER, Johannes A, van der Ven AM. Clinical value of bacteriological examinations of nasal and paranasal mucosa in patients with chronic sinusitis. European Archives of Oto-Rhino-Laryngology. 2001;**258**(5):220-225

[24] AlMutairi D, Kilty SJ. Bacterial biofilms and pathophysiology of chronic rhinosinusitis. Current Opinion in Allergy and Clinical Immunology. 2011;**11**:18-23

[25] Foreman A, Psalitis AJ, Tan LW, Wormald PJ. Characterization of bacterial and fungal biofilms in chronic rhinosinusitis. American Journal of Rhinology and Allergy. 2009;**23**(6):556-561

[26] Ferguson BJ, Stolz DB. Demonstration of biofilm in human bacterial chronic rhinosinusitis. American Journal of Rhinology. 2005;**19**(5):452-457

[27] Kotłowski R, Bernstein CN, Sepehri S, Krause DO. High prevalence of *Escherichia coli* belonging to the B2+D phylogenetic group in inflammatory bowel disease. Gut. 2007;**56**:669-675

[28] Johnson JR, Stell AL, Delavari P, Murray AC, Kuskowski M, Gaastra W. Phylogenetic and pathotypic similarities between *Escherichia coli* isolates from urinary tract infections in dogs and extraintestinal infections in humans. The Journal of Infectious Diseases. 2001;**183**:897-906

[29] Goluszko P, Moseley S, Truong LD, Kaul A, Nowicki S, Nowicki B. Development of experimental model of chronic pyelonephritis with *Escherichia coli* O75:K5:H—bearing Dr fimbriae: Mutation in the dra region prevented tubulointerstitial nephritis. The Journal of Clinical Investigation. 1997;**99**:1-11

[30] Kostakioti M, Hadjifrangiskou M, Hultgren SJ. Bacterial biofilms: Development, dispersal, and therapeutic strategies in the dawn of the postantibiotic era. Cold Spring Harbor Perspectives in Medicine. 2013;**3**(4):1-23

[31] Nowicki B, Vuopio-Varkila J, Viljanen P, Korhonen T, Makela PH.

Fimbrial phase variation and systemic *E. coli* infection studied in mouse peritonitis model. Microbial Pathogen. 1986;**1**:335-347

[32] Nowicki B, Sledzinska A, Samet A, Nowicki S. Pathogenesis of gestational UTI: Urinary obstruction vs. immune adaptation and microbial virulence. BJOG: An International Journal of Obstetrics and Gynaecology. 2011;**118**(2):109-112

[33] Heras B, Totsika M, Peters KM, Paxman JJ, Gee CL, Jarrott RJ, et al. The antigen 43 structure reveals a molecular velcro-like mechanism of autotransporter-mediated bacterial clumping. Proceedings of the National Academy of Sciences of the United States of America. 2014;**111**(1):457-462

[34] Mulvey MA, Lopez-Boado YS, Wilson CL, Roth R, Parks WC, Heuser J, et al. Induction and evasion of host defenses by type 1-piliated uropathogenic *Escherichia coli*. Science. 1998;**282**(5393):1494-1497

[35] Schubert S, Rakin A, Karch H, Carniel E, Heesemann J. Prevalence of the "high-pathogenicity island" of *Yersinia* species among *Escherichia coli* strains that are pathogenic to humans. Infection and Immunity. 1998;**66**:480-485

[36] Hancock V, Ferrières L, Klemm P. The ferric yersiniabactin uptake receptor FyuA is required for efficient biofilm formation by urinary tract infectious *Escherichia coli* in human urine. Microbiology. 2008;**154**(1):167-175

[37] Długaszewska J, Leszczyńska M, Lenkowski M, Tatarska A, Pastusiak T, Szyfter W. The pathophysiological role of bacterial biofilms in chronic sinusitis. European Archives of Oto-Rhino-Laryngology. 2016;**273**:1989-1994

[38] Ramadan HH, Sanclement JA, Thomas JG. Chronic rhinosinusitis and biofilms. Otolaryngology and Head and Neck Surgery. 2005;**132**:414-417

[39] Larson DA, Han JK. Microbiology of sinusitis: Does allergy or endoscopic sinus surgery affect the microbiologic flora? Current Opinion in Otolaryngology and Head and Neck Surgery. 2011;**19**:199-203

[40] Jain R, Waldvogel-Thurlow S, Darveau R, Douglas R. Differences in the paranasal sinuses between germ-free and pathogen-free mice. International Forum of Allergy and Rhinologyis. 2016;**6**(6):631-637

[41] Radtsig EY, Selkova EP, Malygina LV, Lapitskaia AS. The role of respiratory viruses in etiology of rhinosinusitis in the children. Vestnik Otorinolaringologii. 2014;**6**:39-40

[42] Beule AG. Epidemiology of chronic rhinosinusitis, selected risk factors, comorbidities and economic burden. Laryngo-Rhino-Otologie. 2015;**94**(Suppl 1):S1-S23

[43] Kaul A, Goluszko PG, Hart A, Martens M, Pham T, Nowicki S, et al. Rapid cycle changes in density and accessibility of endometrial ligands for *Escherichia coli* Dr fimbriae. Infection and Immunity. 1996;**64**:611-615

[44] Nowicki B, Nowicki S. CD55 as a therapeutic target for steroid hormones: Implications for host pathogen interaction: In: Lambris JD, Holers VM, Ricklin D, editors. Special Issue on Complement Therapeutics, Advances in Experimental Medicine and Biology. Vol. 734. Springer; 2013. pp. 83-96

[45] Nowicki B. Urinary tract infection in pregnant women: Old dogmas and current concepts. Current Infectious Disease Reports. 2002;**4**:529-535

[46] Moulds JM, Nowicki S, Nowicki BJ, Moulds JJ. Human blood groups: Incidental receptors for viruses and

bacteria. Transfusion. 1996;**36**:362-374. Invited review

[47] Nowicki B, Nowicki S, Selvarangan R. Family of *Escherichia coli* Dr adhesins: Decay-accelerating factor receptor recognition and invasiveness. The Journal of Infectious Diseases. 2001;**183**(Suppl 1):S24-S27

[48] Johnson JR, Stell AL. Extended virulence genotypes of *Escherichia coli* strains from patients with urosepsis in relation to phylogeny and host compromise. The Journal of Infectious Diseases. 2000;**181**:261-272

[49] Krawczyk B, Śledzińska A, Szemiako K, Samet A, Nowicki B, Kur J. Characterisation of *Escherichia coli* isolates from the blood of haematological adult patients with bacteraemia: Translocation from gut to blood requires the cooperation of multiple virulence factors. European Journal of Clinical Microbiology and Infectious Diseases. 2015;**34**(6):1135-1143

[50] Szemiako K, Krawczyk B, Samet A, Śledzińska A, Nowicki B, Nowicki S, et al. A subset of two adherence systems, acute pro-inflammatory *pap* genes and invasion coding *dra*, *fim*, or *sfa*, increases the risk of *Escherichia coli* translocation to the bloodstream. European Journal of Clinical Microbiology and Infectious Diseases. 2013;**32**(12):1579-1582

[51] Le Bouguenec C, Archambaud M, Labigne A. Rapid and specific detection of the *pap*, *afa*, and *sfa* adhesin encoding operons in uropathogenic *Escherichia coli* strains by polymerase chain reaction. Journal of Clinical Microbiology. 1992;**30**:1189-1193

[52] Krawczyk B, Samet A, Leibner J, Śledzińska A, Kur J. Evaluation of a PCR melting profile technique for bacterial strain differentiation. Journal of Clinical Microbiology. 2006;**44**:2327-2332

[53] Clermont O, Bonacorsi S, Bingen E. Rapid and simple determination of the *Escherichia coli* phylogenetic group. Applied and Environmental Microbiology. 2000;**66**:4555-4558

[54] Adamus-Białek W, Wojtasik A, Majchrzak M, Sosnowski M, Parniewski P. (CGG)4 based PCR as a novel tool for discrimination of uropathogenic *Escherichia coli* strains: Comparison with enterobacterial repetitive intergenic consensus PCR. Journal of Clinical Microbiology. 2009;**47**:3937-3944

[55] Johnson JR, Brown JJ, Carlino UB, Russo TA. Colonization with and acquisition of uropathogenic *Escherichia coli* as revealed by polymerase chain reaction-based detection. The Journal of Infectious Diseases. 1998;**177**:1120-1124

[56] Krawczyk B, Śledzińska A, Piekarska A, Hellmann A, Kur J. Recurrent bowel-blood translocations of *Escherichia coli w*ith the unique virulence characteristics over three-year period in the patient with acute myeloid leukaemia—Case report. Journal of Applied Genetics. 2017;**58**(3):415-418

[57] Nowak-Zaleska A, Wieczór M, Czub J, Nierzwicki Ł, Kotłowski R, Mikucka A, et al. Correlation between the number of Pro-Ala repeats in the EmrA homologue of Acinetobacter baumannii and resistance to netilmicin, tobramycin, imipenem and ceftazidime. Journal of Global Antimicrobial Resistance. 2016;**7**:145-149

[58] Mobley HLT, Alteri CJ. Development of a vaccine against *Escherichia coli* urinary tract infections. Pathogens. 2016;**5**(1):1

Chapter 5

Rhinosinusitis: How Common Are Anatomical Variations Responsible?

Shrikant Phatak and Richa Agrawal

Abstract

The term rhinosinusitis is defined as inflammation of nose and paranasal sinuses characterised by nasal blockage, nasal discharge, post-nasal drip, facial pain, pressure and reduction/loss of smell with corresponding endoscopic appearance and CT scan changes. The combined term is more apt than individual rhinitis or sinusitis as it is unusual for having sinus inflammation alone in the absence of nasal inflammation. The disease occurs due to obstruction in the key area, i.e., the osteomeatal complex (OMC). This chapter discusses anatomical variations responsible for the blockage of OMC leading to rhinosinusitis. Nasal endoscopic findings and radiological features depicting these variations are discussed in detail.

Keywords: rhinosinusitis, anatomical variations, osteomeatal complex, nasal endoscopy, imaging

1. Introduction

The approach of an otolaryngologist towards the management of sinusitis has changed significantly after the development of endoscopes and imaging techniques. Both these modalities help in thorough understanding of surgical anatomy and prominent anatomical variations of nose and paranasal sinuses (PNS).

Diagnostic nasal endoscopy (DNE) and imaging are complimentary to each other as small polyps in the areas of sinus ostia can often be missed in a CT scan. CT scan is still the mainstay of diagnosis for inflammatory sinonasal pathology because this displays the anatomy in a perspective that is useful to the surgeon [1]. The coronal plane, in particular, is considered as a map for assessing the anatomy that varies significantly even between both sides in the same individual. CT scan gives complete information about normal anatomy, anatomical variations, the extent of disease, and relation of sinuses to adjoining vital structures such as orbit and intracranial areas. Hence, the surgeon should master the normal surgical as well as radiological anatomy and probable anatomical variations for successful surgical outcomes.

2. Surgical anatomy

Nasal cavity is divided into right and left halves by the nasal septum. The right and left nasal cavities are often considered as mirror image; however, this may not be the case [2]. In the lateral nasal wall there lie openings of maxillary, frontal, ethmoid, and sphenoid sinuses. The lateral nasal wall is convoluted and has got three turbinates: superior, middle, and inferior turbinate. Sometimes there can also be a supreme turbinate. Beneath each turbinate lies the corresponding meatus, namely superior meatus, middle meatus, and inferior meatus, respectively. Superior meatus is confined to the posterior third of lateral wall, the middle meatus about two thirds of the length, and inferior meatus extends along the whole length of the lateral wall. Superior meatus has opening of posterior ethmoids, while the sphenoid opens in the sphenoethmoidal recess. Middle meatus harbours the opening of frontal, maxillary, and anterior ethmoidal sinuses. The nasolacrimal duct opens in the inferior meatus.

The superior and middle turbinate are the part of ethmoid bone, while inferior turbinate is a separate bone. Middle turbinate is the most important landmark for the sinus surgery, and therefore, its attachments are important. The anterior portion lies in the sagittal plane and inserts into the lateral border of cribriform plate of ethmoidal bone. The central portion rotates in the coronal plane and is attached to the lamina papyracea. This part is known as basal or ground lamella of middle turbinate. The ground lamella separates anterior ethmoidal cells from the posterior ethmoidal cells. The posterior portion of the middle turbinate runs in the horizontal plane and is attached to the perpendicular plate of palatine bone.

2.1 Paranasal sinuses

The sinuses are arranged in pairs in relation to each nasal cavity, comprising two groups: anterior and posterior. The maxillary, frontal, and anterior ethmoids form the anterior group and these drain into the middle meatus. The posterior ethmoids and sphenoid form the posterior group which drain into superior meatus and sphenoethmoidal recess, respectively. The maxillary sinus exists at birth as small but definitive cavity adjacent to the middle meatus and it gradually enlarges with the eruption of primary dentition, and by the age of 7th year, it reaches the level of nasal floor. It attains the maximum dimension by the age of 21 years, when its floor lies 4–5 mm below the floor of nose [3]. The natural ostium is located in the superior aspect of the medial wall of the sinus and drains into hiatus semilunaris. Frontal sinus is rudimentary at birth and it reaches the level of orbital roof at the age of 9 years and its development is completed by 20 years. There is minimal development of sphenoid sinus until 3 years of age after this sphenoid sinus begins to pneumatise the sphenoid bone. There is a great variation in the extent of pneumatisation of the sphenoid sinus. It may be present as a small pit in a predominantly nonpneumatised sphenoid bone—Conchal Type. It may extend up to the anterior wall of sella turcica—Presellar type. It may pneumatise the entire sphenoid body below and behind the sella turcica so that the pituitary forms distinct bulge in its posterosuperior wall—Sellar Type [4]. Ethmoidal sinuses are the most complex of the sinuses and they are present at birth and attain adult size by the age of 12 years.

2.2 Osteomeatal complex

The term OMC is used to refer collectively the maxillary sinus ostium, ethmoid infundibulum, hiatus semilunaris, middle meatus, frontal recess, ethmoidal bulla, and uncinate process. It describes the final drainage pathway of the anterior group of sinuses.

2.3 Mucociliary clearance

Secretions of nose and sinuses form a sheet called mucous blanket. Mucous blanket consists of a superficial mucus layer, floating on the top of cilia which constantly beat like a conveyer belt towards the nasopharynx; the inspired bacterial viruses and dust particles are entrapped on the mucous blanket and carried to the nasopharynx to be swallowed. Hampering of the mucociliary mechanism leads to the stasis of secretions and subsequent sinusitis [5].

2.4 Anatomical variations

Variation in anatomy is a rule than an exception. Nature has customised different anatomies for every individual. Therefore, one must be aware of these possible variations before any surgical interventions. The major consequences of these anatomical variations are narrowing of the infundibulum.

Air in the nose and PNS act as natural contrast, so CT scan in bone and soft tissue windows is sufficient to diagnose anatomical variations and pathology in most of the cases of chronic rhinosinusitis (CRS). Here, a brief account of radiological images of anatomical variations and corresponding nasal endoscopic findings is discussed.

- DNS

  It is the commonest anatomical variation. Deviation of posterior nasal septum causes CRS by creating pressure and air flow changes within the maxillary sinuses [6] (**Figures 1** and **2**). Septal spur causes turbulence in airflow leading to polyp formation.

- Concha bullosa

  It is pneumatisation of middle turbinate involving its inferior bullous portion, and it may be bilateral [7, 8]. Large concha causes significant obstruction of nose. Such patients present with sinogenic headaches or chronic sinusitis. Sometimes there can be pneumatisation of lamina of middle turbinate known as lamellar concha.

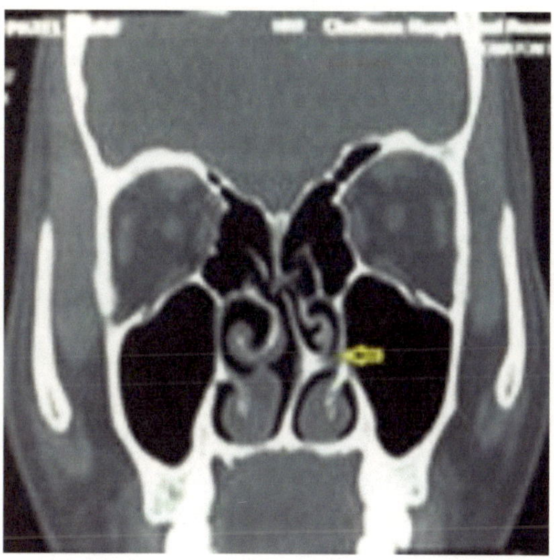

Figure 1.
CT showing sharp spur impinging middle turbinate.

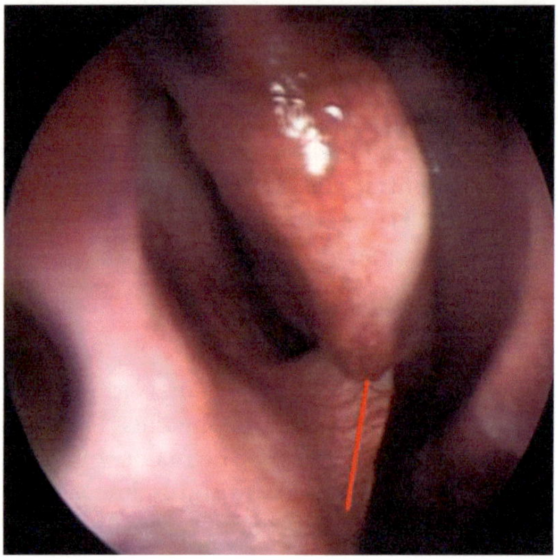

Figure 2.
Endoscopic picture showing spur impacting middle turbinate in left nasal cavity.

A paradoxical bent of middle turbinate is defined as turbinate having convexity towards the lateral nasal wall. This leads to narrowing of infundibulum [9–11] (**Figures 3** and **4**).

- Pneumatisation of superior turbinate- (**Figure 5**)

- Uncinate process

Can be medially bent uncinate process (**Figures 6** and **7**) or pneumatised uncinate process (**Figures 8** and **9**). Sometimes the uncinate can protrude anterior-inferior to middle turbinate, giving the impression of two middle turbinates [12].

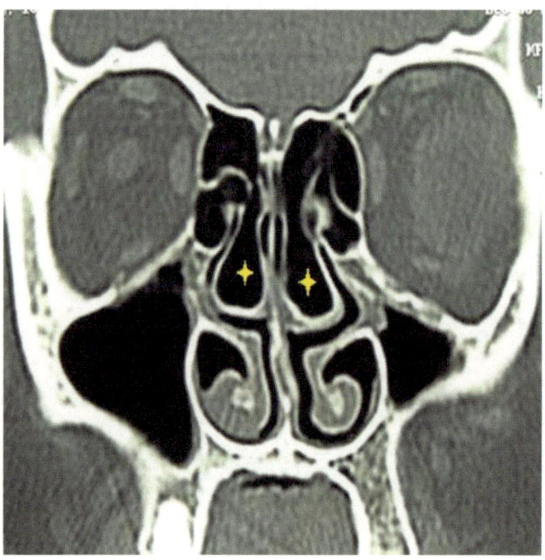

Figure 3.
CT PNS showing bilateral concha bullosa.

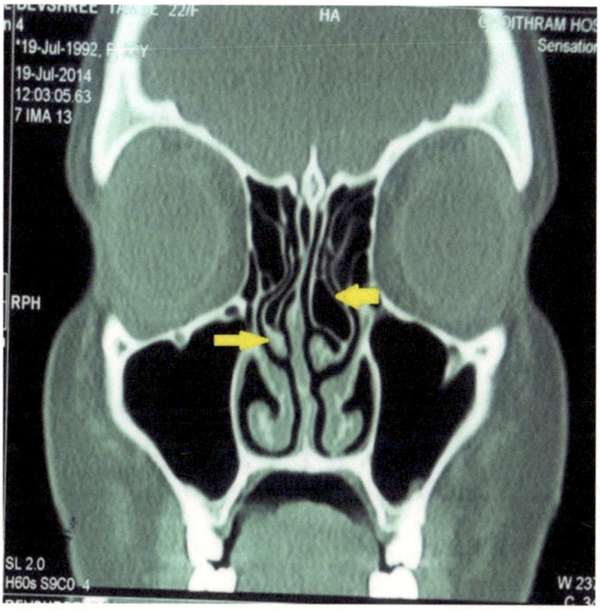

Figure 4.
CT PNS showing bilateral paradoxical middle turbinate with right lamellar concha.

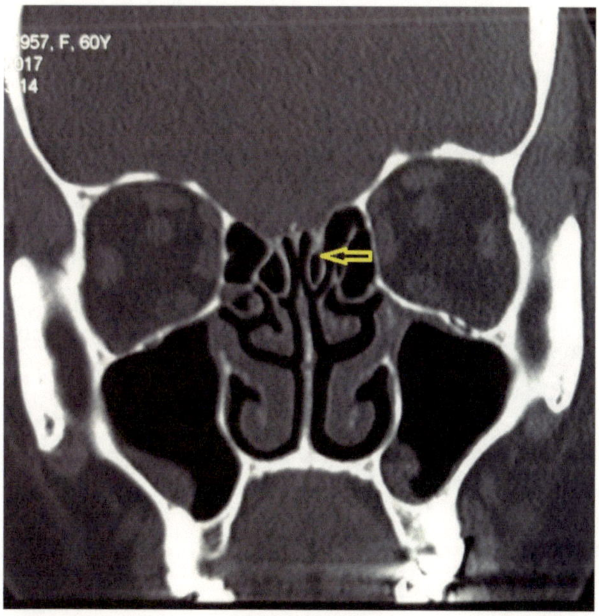

Figure 5.
CT PNS coronal cuts showing pneumatisation of superior turbinate.

- Big agar

Agar cells are usually pneumatised from the frontal recess. Extensively pneumatised agger nasi cells will narrow the frontal sinus drainage pathway leading to frontal sinusitis [13]. Agger nasi cells are closely related to lacrimal sac and are separated from the latter by thin lacrimal bone. This bone may also be naturally dehiscent leading to spread of infection and subsequent dacryocystitis (**Figures 10** and **11**).

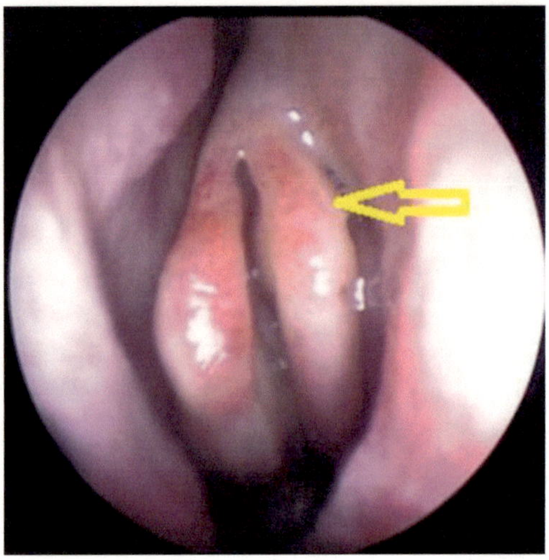

Figure 6.
DNE showing medially bent uncinate process.

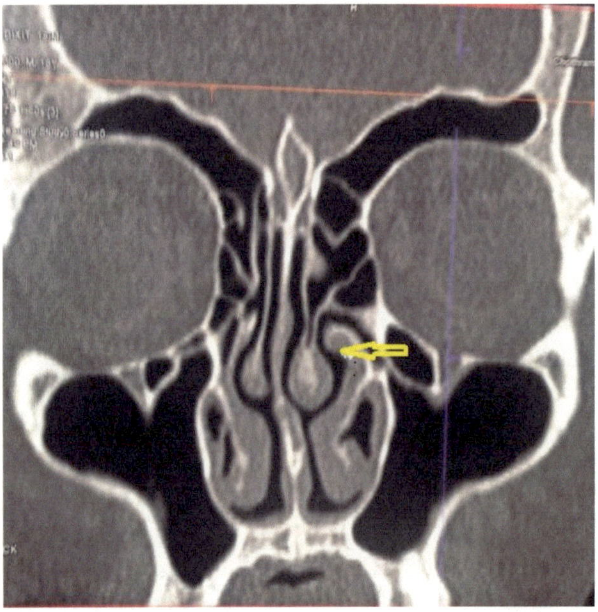

Figure 7.
CT showing thick and medially bent uncinate process.

- Haller cell

The presence of infraorbital ethmoidal cells can obstruct the drainage pathway of the maxillary sinus and also increase the risk of orbital injury during ethmoidectomy (**Figure 12**).

- Onodi cell

It is insinuation of posterior ethmoid air cell between optic nerve and sphenoid sinus. It is associated with increased risk of injury with optic nerve or carotid artery during functional endoscopic sinus surgery (FESS) [14] (**Figure 13**).

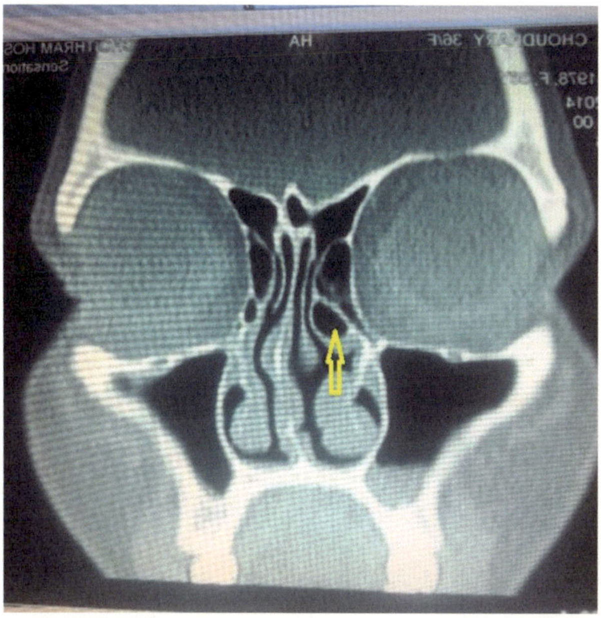

Figure 8.
CT showing pneumatised uncinate process on left side.

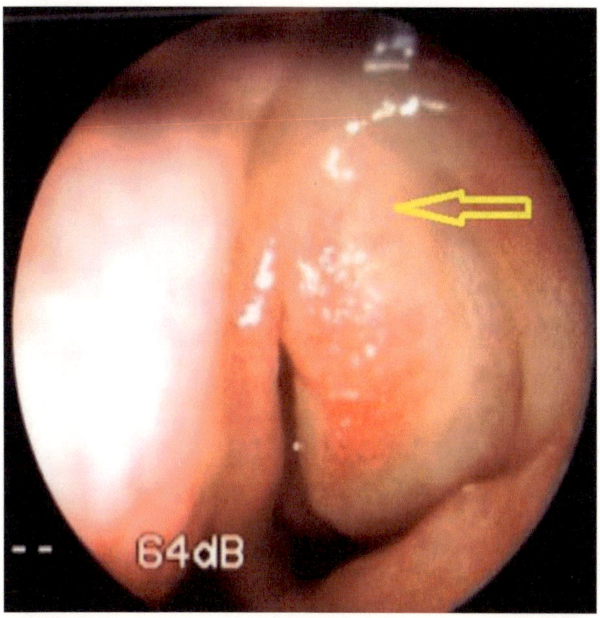

Figure 9.
Endoscopy showing pneumatised uncinate process.

- Accessory ostia

Maxillary sinus drains through the natural ostia and the presence of accessory ostia does not play a role in its physiologic drainage. Rather, it leads to mucous recirculation and CRS [15] (**Figures 14** and **15**).

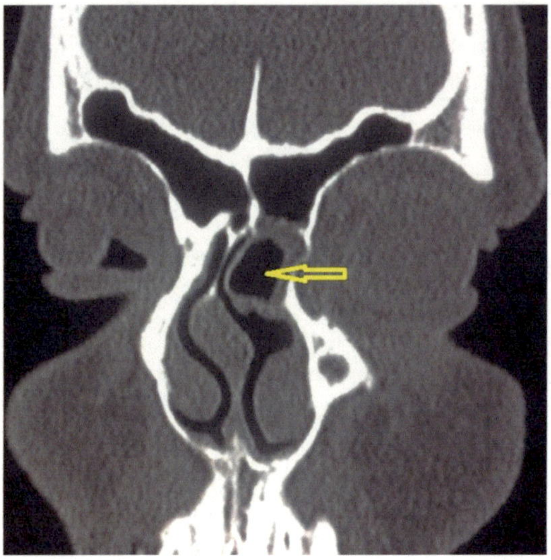

Figure 10.
CT PNS showing big agar on left side. Note that frontal sinuses are still clear.

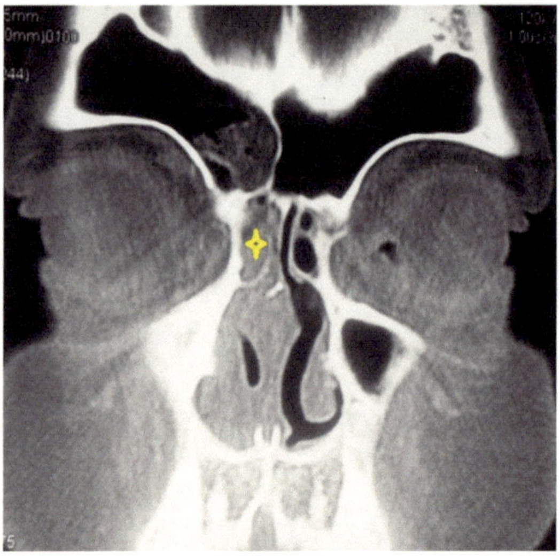

Figure 11.
CT PNS showing infected agar on right side with haziness in right frontal sinus.

- Hypoplasia/agenesis of maxillary sinus

According to Bolger and Parsons, maxillary sinus hypoplasia can be classified into three types:

Type I—There is mild decrease in maxillary sinus volume with normal uncinate and normal ethmoid infundibulum.

Type II—There is mild-to-moderate reduction in volume of maxillary sinus combined with CT evidence of an absent or hypoplastic uncinate process and an absent or poorly defined ethmoid infundibulum due to uncinate process being fused with the inferomedial wall of the orbit.

Type III—Maxillary sinus is primarily absent. Ethmoid infundibulum and uncinate process are absent [16].

In our case, there was type III maxillary sinus hypoplasia (**Figures 16** and **17**).

DOI: http://dx.doi.org/10.5772/intechopen.83689

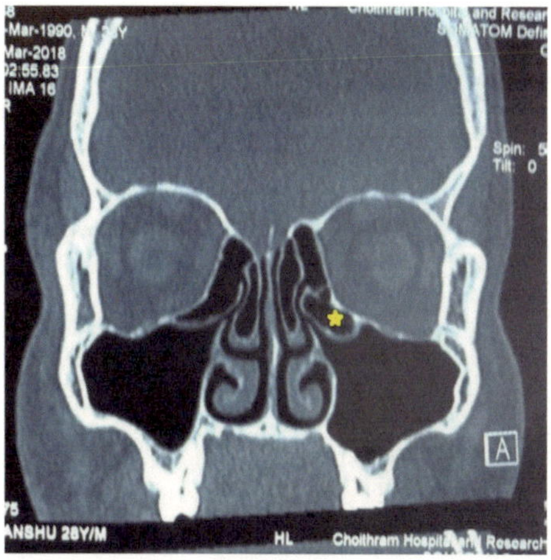

Figure 12.
CT PNS showing Haller cell on left side with narrowing of infundibulum. Sinuses are still clear.

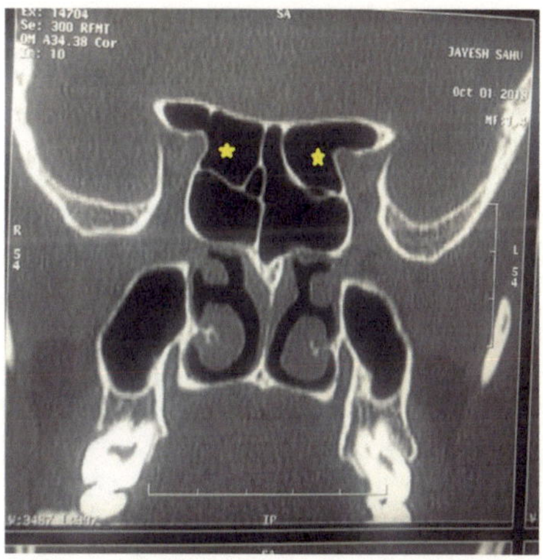

Figure 13.
Coronal section of PNS showing bilateral Onodi cell.

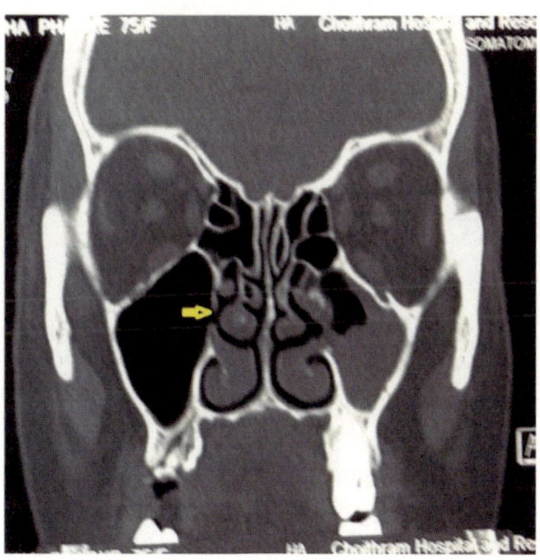

Figure 14.
CT PNS showing accessory ostia on right with clear maxillary. On the contrary, opposite sinus is hazy.

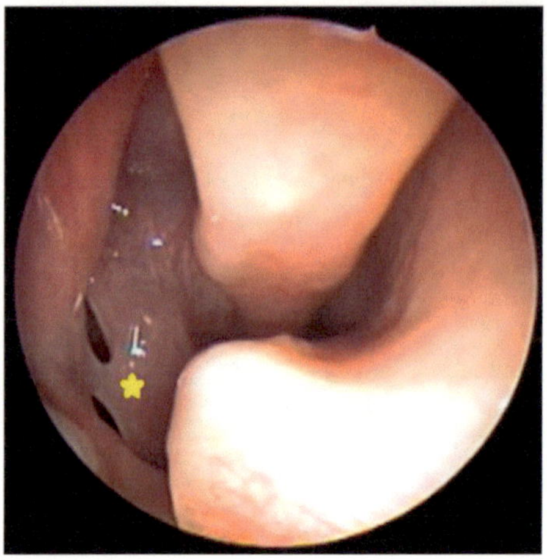

Figure 15.
Endoscopy showing two accessory ostia.

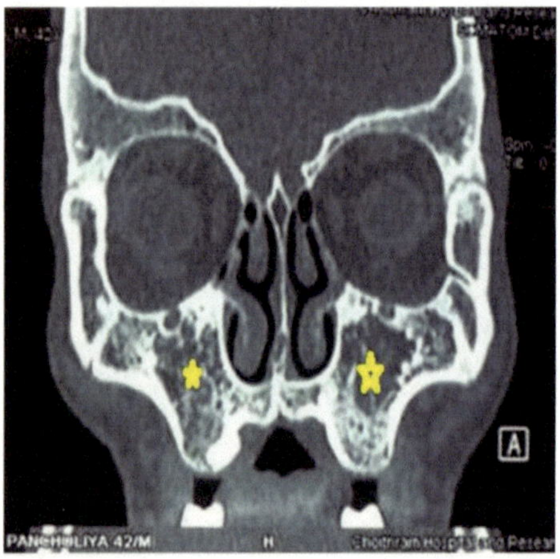

Figure 16.
CT showing hypoplasia of bilateral maxillary sinus.

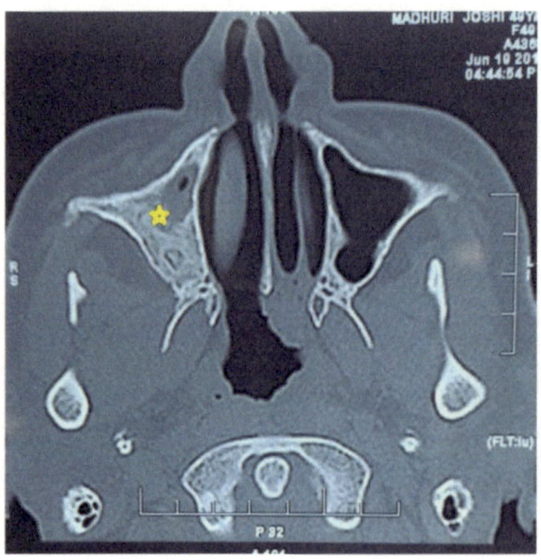

Figure 17.
CT (axial section) agenesis of right maxillary sinus.

- Pneumatisation of septum (**Figure 18**)

The septum may be pneumatised as a result of extension of an aerated crista galli or anterior extension of the sphenoid sinus.

- Persistent adenoids

Adenoids are present at birth and usually regress by 12–14 years of age. With advent of CT PNS, it is now clear that adenoids may persist even after adolescence. In our case, adenoids persisted till 56 years of age; this patient too had presented with CRS (**Figures 19** and **20**).

There is evidence that the adenoid provides a reservoir of bacteria that may be a pathogenic factor in the development of CRS. Biofilms overlying the adenoid pad may prevent antibiotic therapy from clearing the infection. Adenoidectomy surgically removes this reservoir for chronic infection [17].

- KEROS classification (**Figures 21–24**)

Depending upon the depth of olfactory fossa Keros classification is as follows:

KEROS type I—Depth of olfactory fossa is 1–3 mm.

KEROS type II—Depth of olfactory fossa is 4–7 mm.

KEROS type III—Depth of olfactory fossa is 8–14 mm.

Type I is the safest while type III has high chances of skull base injury during ethmoidectomy.

Asymmetry of ethmoid roof on both sides of the same patient is not uncommon. Hence, the surgeon should read CT thoroughly before any surgical intervention.

- Low anterior ethmoidal artery

Anterior ethmoidal artery is an important landmark in sinus surgery. The anterior ethmoidal artery is seen as a classical breaking of the medial orbital wall. The artery may lie close to the skull base or may cross low within anterior ethmoid in which case the orbitocranial canal with its bony mesentery is clearly seen [4] (**Figure 25**). If the anterior ethmoidal notch is abutting the lateral lamella or the fovea ethmoidalis, the artery is considered protected during functional

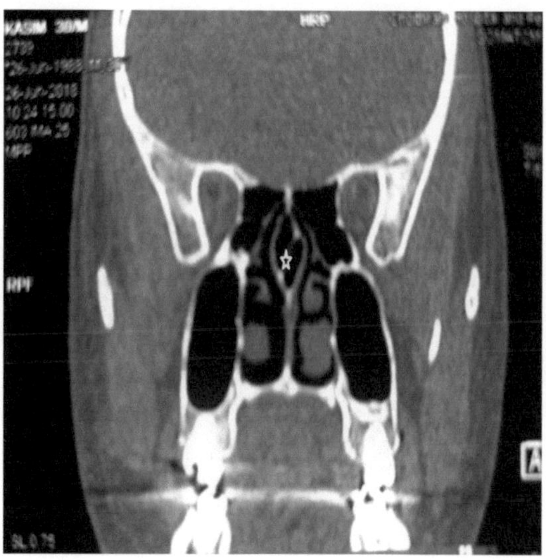

Figure 18.
CT showing septal pneumatisation.

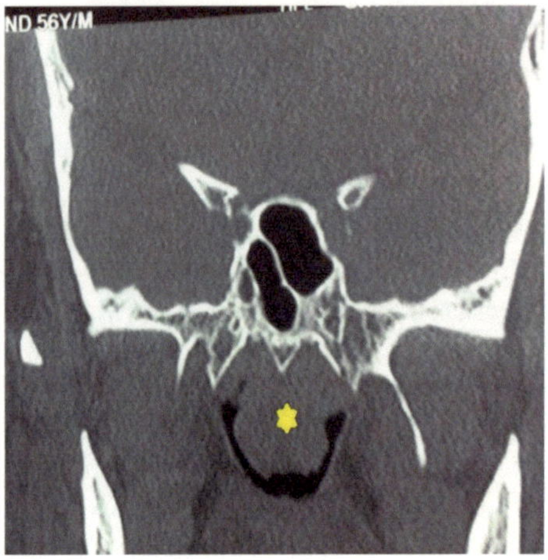

Figure 19.
CT showing persistent adenoids in a 56-year-old patient.

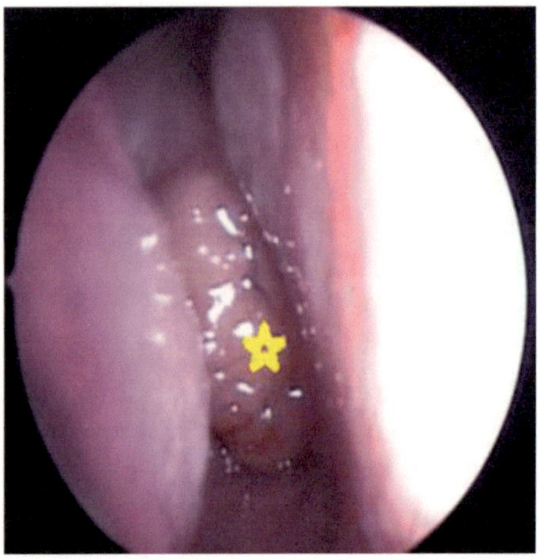

Figure 20.
Endoscopic showing persistent adenoids.

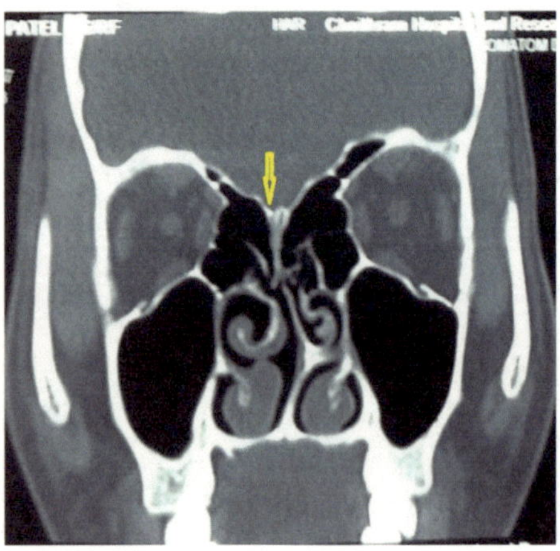

Figure 21.
CT showing KEROS type I.

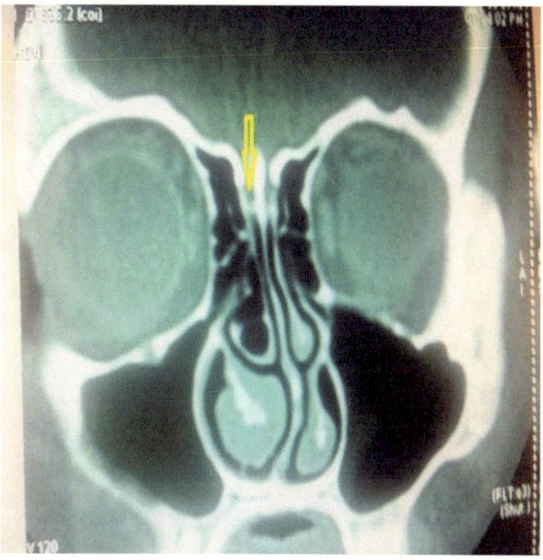

Figure 22.
CT showing KEROS type II.

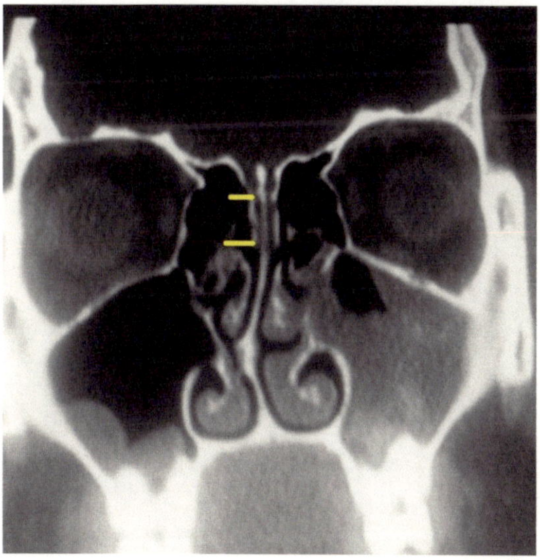

Figure 23.
CT showing KEROS type III.

endoscopic sinus surgery as it is as the level of the skull base. If a supraorbital cell is seen above the anterior ethmoidal notch, or if the artery is located below the skull base, it is considered at risk [18, 19].

- Dehiscent lamina papyracea (**Figure 26**)

Natural dehiscence in lamina papyracea will result in prolapse of orbital contents into the nasal cavity. The defects allow easy damage to the orbit during FESS and also increase the risk of orbital contents being drawn into the microdebrider.

The incidence of anatomical variations responsible for CRS in decreasing order of their frequency is as follows:

Deviated nasal septum—the commonest anatomical variation with 69% incidence.

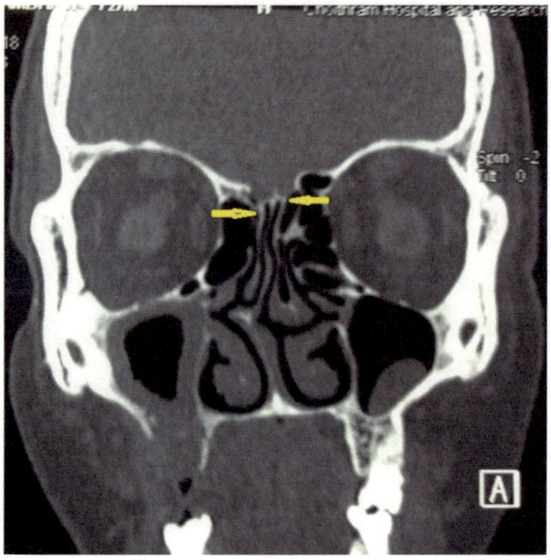

Figure 24.
CT showing asymmetrical ethmoidal roof.

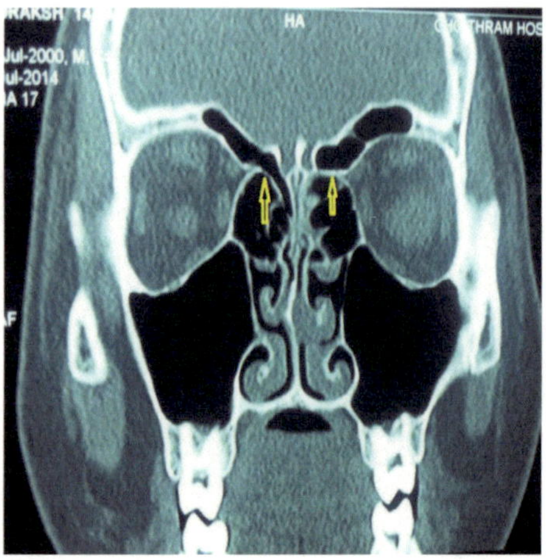

Figure 25.
CT showing low bilateral low anterior ethmoidal artery.

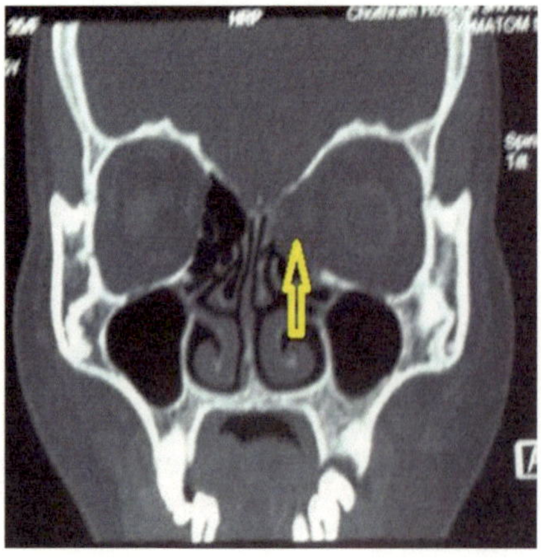

Figure 26.
CT PNS (coronal view) showing dehiscent lamina with fat prolapse on left side.

DOI: http://dx.doi.org/10.5772/intechopen.83689

Concha—24%.

Unilateral concha was seen in 13%, while bilateral concha was seen in 11% cases.

Big agar—12%.

Pneumatised or medially bent uncinate—8%.

Accessory ostia—6%.

Septal pneumatisation—5%.

Onodi cell—4%.

Haller cell—3%.

Hypoplasia of maxillary sinus with dehiscent lamina was seen in less than 2% of cases.

3. Conclusion

The presence of anatomical variations in nose and sinuses is frequently seen on imaging in patients with CRS. It is observed that the presence of more than one variation increases the probability of sinus infections. However, it is not the rule as there can be clear sinuses even with multiple anatomical variations.

Acknowledgements

Dr. Sunil Chandiwal. Director Medical Services. Choithram Hospital & Research Centre. Indore, India. Source of funding: None.

Conflict of interest

None.

Appendices and nomenclature

OMC	osteomeatal complex
PNS	paranasal sinuses
DNE	diagnostic nasal endoscopy
CRS	chronic rhinosinusitis
FESS	functional endoscopic sinus surgery

Author details

Shrikant Phatak* and Richa Agrawal
Department of ENT, Choithram Hospital and Research Centre, Indore, India

*Address all correspondence to: phatakshrikant2@gmail.com

References

[1] Shankar L, Evans K. An Atlas of Imaging of the Paranasal Sinuses. 2nd ed. Lippincott Williams & Wilkins; 2009. p. 28

[2] Kirtane MV, de Souza CE. Rhinology and Endoscopic Skull Base Surgery. Thieme; 2013. p. 8

[3] Mclay K, Maran AGD, Dale BAB, Cowan DL, Kerr AIG. Logan Turner's. Diseases of the Nose, Throat and Ear. 9th ed. John Wright & Sons; 1982. pp. 9-11

[4] Bradoo R. Anatomical Principal of Endoscopic Sinus Surgery: A Step by Step Approach. 1st ed. Jaypee Brothers Medical Publishers; 2016. p.78

[5] Dhingra PL, Dhingra S. Disease of Ear, Nose and Throat & Head and Neck Surgery. 6th ed. Elsevier; 2014. pp. 140-141

[6] Hasan OA, Hassan MA, Fawzy EK, Maarouf AM. Anatomical variations of nasal structures in chronic rhinosinusitis as detected by computed tomography scan. The Egyptian Journal of Hospital Medicine. 2017;**68**(3):1390-1394

[7] Kantarci M, Karasen RM, Alper F, et al. Remarkable anatomic variations in paranasal sinus region and their clinical importance. European Journal of Radiology. 2004;**50**:296-302

[8] Beale TJ, Madani G, Morley SJ. Imaging of the paranasal sinuses and nasal cavity: Normal anatomy and clinically relevant anatomical variants. Seminars in Ultrasound, CT, and MR. 2009;**30**:2-16

[9] Azila A, Irfan M, Rohaizan Y, et al. The prevalence of anatomical variations in osteomeatal unit in patients with chronic rhinosinusitis. The Medical Journal of Malaysia. 2011;**66**:191-194

[10] Fadda GL, Rosso S, Aversa S, et al. Multiparametric statistical correlations between paranasal sinus anatomic variations and chronic rhinosinusitis. Acta Otorhinolaryngologica Italica. 2012;**32**:244-251

[11] Nouraei SA, Elisay AR, Dimarco A, et al. Variations in paranasal sinus anatomy: Implications for the pathophysiology of chronic rhinosinusitis and safety of endoscopic sinus surgery. Journal of Otolaryngology—Head & Neck Surgery. 2009;**38**:32-37

[12] Polavaram R, Devaiah AK, Sakai O, Shapshay SM. Anatomic variants and pearls-functional endoscopic sinus surgery. Otolaryngologic Clinics of North America. 2004;**37**:221-242

[13] Brunner E, Jacobs JB, Shpizner BA, Lebowitz RA, Holliday RA. Role of agar nasi cell in chronic frontal sinusitis. The Annals of Otology, Rhinology, and Laryngology. 1996;**105**(5):694-700

[14] Tomovic S, Esmaeili A, Chan NJ, et al. High-resolution computed tomography analysis of the prevalence of Onodi cells. Laryngoscope. 2012;**122**:1470-1473

[15] Yanagisawa E, Yanagisawa K. Endoscopic view of recirculation phenomenon of the maxillary sinus. Ear, Nose, & Throat Journal. 1997;**76**:196-198

[16] Bolger WE, Butzin CA, Parsons DS. Paranasal sinus bony anatomic variation and mucosal abnormalities: CT analysis for endoscopic sinus surgery. Laryngoscope. 1991;**101**:56-64

[17] Arthur WW, Shapiro NL, Bhattacharya N. Chronic rhinosinusitis in children: What are treatment options? Immunology and Allergy Clinics of North America. 2009;**29**(4):705-717

[18] Kirtane MV. Endoscopic Endonasal Surgery: Sinuses and Beyond. 1st ed. Jaypee Brothers Medical Publishers. 2015. p. 9

[19] Simmen D, Raghavan U, Briner HR, et al. The surgeon's view of the anterior ethmoid artery. Clinical Otolaryngology. 2006;**31**(3):187-191

Chapter 6

Refractory Rhinosinusitis

Yi-Tsen Lin and Te-Huei Yeh

Abstract

Various factors have been proposed to be related to refractory chronic rhinosinusitis (CRS). Treatment for refractory CRS is challenging for ear, nose, and throat (ENT) surgeons. The aim of the study was to determine the clinical features associated with the severity of CRS that may necessitate revision surgery by eliminating the bias of the surgeon's technique using standardizing surgical procedures. Sinus wall thickness and blood eosinophilia, which may represent the depth of inflammation in CRS, are associated with the need for revision surgery. We found that, when the thickness of the posterolateral maxillary sinus wall is more than 3.03 mm, there is an increased probability for a need for revision surgery. CRS patients with thickened sinus walls were found to have poorer outcomes. Further research is needed in order to justify this type of surgical procedure for CRS.

Keywords: refractory, chronic rhinosinusitis, inflammation, osteitis, eosinophilia

1. Introduction

The sinonasal organ plays an important role in the human respiratory system, as this organ consistently encounters external irritants and is therefore one of the most frequently inflamed sites in the human body [1]. Inflammation may begin as an infectious process (acute rhinosinusitis), and, if the symptoms persist without resolution, it can lead to inflammatory consequences (chronic rhinosinusitis (CRS)) [2]. CRS is one of the most prevalent chronic diseases in modern society and is defined as the presence of more than one nasal symptom (mucopurulent drainage, nasal congestion, facial pain-pressure-fullness, and decreased sense of smell) and a documentation of inflammation for more than 12 weeks [3]. It is a heterogeneous, multifactorial disease with multiple distinct factors, including genetic, infectious, immune, anatomic, allergic, and inflammatory components [2]. The goal of CRS therapy is maximal medical treatment including oral and topical antibiotics, nasal steroids, systemic steroids, antihistamines, and saline irrigations. Functional endoscopic sinus surgery (FESS) is indicated if medical therapy fails [4].

The safety and efficacy of FESS for CRS have been strongly supported by meta-analyses from both large outcome studies and cohort studies. Improvement in both disease-specific and generic quality of life and objective measures have been demonstrated for the efficacy of FESS; however, across long-term follow-up, there is a 10–20% revision rate, which is considered to be refractory CRS [5]. Refractory CRS is defined by failure to stabilize after surgery and treatment with antibiotics, saline rinses, and topical steroid and has become a significant issue for ENT surgeons [6]. Predicting surgical outcome is crucial for evaluating the severity of CRS preoperatively, and the severity of CRS is usually defined by several factors. Temporally, the duration and frequency of symptoms and signs of CRS patients cannot be precisely correlated. Spatially, the Lund-Mackay (L-M) score, which is based on CT images, is the most frequently used method to evaluate the severity of CRS; nevertheless, the L-M score represents only a snapshot of the condition [7]. A swift change in mucosal swelling is frequently observed during the subacute stage of sinusitis. Other parameters should be considered in order to define the severity of CRS and more accurately predict its prognosis.

Various factors are related to refractory CRS, including mucociliary dysfunction, the presence of mucosal biofilm, peripheral eosinophil count, mucosal eosinophilia, acute postoperative infection, ASA triad, cystic fibrosis, osteitis, hyperreactive airway, inhaled allergen, and experience of the performing surgeon [8–12]. It is important to find a simple way to evaluate the severity of CRS in order to identify an accurate prognosis for patients and determine which patients may need long-term medical treatment. The aim of the study was to determine the clinical features related to the severity of CRS that would necessitate revision surgery, by carefully eliminating surgeon bias using standardizing surgical procedures.

2. Standardization of surgical procedure and treatment protocol

The first consideration of this study was to select appropriate patients in order to exclude the congenitally influential factor of heterogeneity of CRS. The next consideration was to standardize the preoperative treatment, surgical procedure, and postoperative follow-up protocol. Over the past 10 years, we have developed a standardized surgical procedure and treatment protocol. Preoperatively, the referral doctor administers optimal medical treatment to the patient; if that does not occur, our clinics will administer the treatment. If treatment fails, surgery is suggested. Preoperative medication is not given for at least 2 weeks, if acute exacerbation was not noted before surgery. Some patients are given a loose schedule of intranasal steroid spray, but oral antibiotics are not given regularly.

Other information are also collected during the preoperative visit: age, gender, asthma, nasal polyps, allergic rhinitis, obstructive sleep apnea, diabetes, smoking status, gastroesophageal reflux disease, prior FESS history, and Samter's triad. For the surgical procedure, the objects of FESS include several folds: to clear out the occluded ostium by correcting the anatomical flaw of bottleneck of draining pathway for diseased sinus, to decrease inflammatory load by removing developed polyps or swollen mucosa which was filled with inflammatory milieu, and to clean out entrapped discharge from deep-seated recess which contained inflammation-inducing materials. Based on the principles described above, we developed eight complete steps to perform standard FESS:

1. Middle turbinate trimming: This procedure is used instead of medial fracture in order to expose the posterior margin of uncinate process and hiatus semilunaris.

2. Uncinectomy: The first step of ethmoidectomy is to properly remove the uncinate process. It can be antegrade, with a sickle knife, or retrograde, by using backbiting forceps, until the superiorly agger nasi cell, and frontal recess and inferiorly the natural ostium of maxillary sinus are identified.

3. Enlargement of the natural ostium of maxillary sinus: By removing the mucosa of posterior fontanelle, the accessory ostium can be identified during this step. Pathologic tissue in the maxillary sinus is removed, and irrigation by normal saline is frequently applied.

4. Removal of the bony wall of the ethmoid bulla: Identifying the basal lamella of the middle turbinate. The retrobullar recess and suprabullar cells are exposed. It is important to expose and identify lamina papyracea in order to delineate the lateral margin of the ethmoid cavity.

5. Removal of the basal lamella at the medial inferior site: In order to enter posterior ethmoid sinus space safely, the middle turbinate insertion is not destabilized. When entering posterior ethmoid space, the superior turbinate and skull base are identified by carefully removing the ethmoid bony septum of the posterior ethmoid sinuses.

6. Opening of the sphenoid sinus, if necessary: The sphenoid sinus is not frequently involved in CRS. If necessary, remove the inferior third of superior turbinate in order to easily find the natural ostium of sphenoid sinus. Irrigation or removing polypoid mucosa surround the ostium is sufficient for most patients.

7. Removal of the bony partitions along the skull base: After identifying the skull base at the posterior ethmoid roof, its is safe to remove the partitions anteriorly to reach the bony indentation of the anterior ethmoid artery (AEA), which is the most important landmark to manage frontal recess. The AEA is a landmark ("Nike" logo-shaped curve) and may be buried inside a bony canal in patients with well-pneumatized anterior ethmoid sinuses; it could be mesenteric. This space is complicated by various possible suprabullar or frontobullar cells and is a challenging step for beginners.

8. Cleaning frontal sinus-draining route: Using the 45-degree endoscope, mark the anatomic landmark of AEA posteriorly and agger nasi or frontoethmoid cells anteriorly; the frontal sinus-draining route is frequently buried in the complicated anterior ethmoid cell system. There may be anteriorly, posteriorly, medially, and laterally located ethmoid air cells; it is important to identify the boundary of ethmoid cavity laterally to the lamina papyracea, medially to the middle turbinate concha, and superiorly along the skull base. The frontal sinus will be safely opened.

Postoperative care includes regularly follow-up for at least 6 months using optimal antibiotic treatment, including low-dose macrolide for 2 months and nasal steroids, as well as routine saline nasal douching plus adjuvant of gentamicin for at least 3 months.

3. Patient selection, radiographic evaluation, and statistical analyses

We reviewed the medical records of 243 patients who received bilateral FESS in our department by the same senior surgeon of a tertiary referral hospital from September 2010 to August 2011. Computed tomography (CT) of paranasal sinuses was performed in all patients at most 2 months prior to surgery. Other preoperative evaluations included hematologic examination the day before surgery. Patients with known systemic diseases or malignancies were excluded, such as diabetes mellitus, asthma, or other immunocompromised diseases. Forty-eight CRS patients who received revised sinus surgery during this period were recruited; 21 of these patients received surgery by the same surgeon, and the other 27 patients received surgery from different surgeons. Among the 21 patients, patients with no previous sinus CT scan available for comparison were excluded. Among the 27 patients, we excluded the patients who received previous Caldwell-Luc procedures. Nine patients were assigned to Group A (primary and revised surgery by the same senior surgeon), 17 patients were assigned to Group B (previously operated on by other surgeons), and 30 control patients were assigned to Group C who received primary FESS surgery during the same period and were followed up for at least 3 years without revision surgery. Group D included 30 control patients with head and neck CT scan from parotid surgery without notified sinonasal problems. Hematologic examination was evaluated for Group D patients 1 day prior to surgery. The flow chart of patient selection is shown in **Figure 1**. The clinical information including the result of bacterial culture and pathology to evaluate eosinophilic rhinosinusitis, with or without asthma and ImmunoCAP Specific IgE blood test, were also collected for further analysis.

The extent of paranasal sinus mucosal disease was evaluated by using the L-M staging system [7]. Sinus wall thickness was measured in coronal view of the sinus CT. The posterolateral wall of maxillary sinus, para-crista galli level (around the lateral lamella) of the ethmoid sinus, and the anterior clinoid level of sphenoid sinus were measured as the representative thickness of each sinus wall (**Figure 2**). All CT studies were performed by 64 multidetector-row CTs (LightSpeed VCT, GE Medical Systems). Contiguous axial 1.2-mm-thick slices were obtained through the maxillofacial bones, and images were reconstructed with soft tissue and bone reconstruction algorithms; 3.0-mm-thick coronal and sagittal reformatted images were obtained per our institutional protocol. All CT measurements were made on bone algorithm reconstructed and bone-windowed images (W:2000, L:500) using an independent workstation. The measurements were repeated by two independent otolaryngologists. In detail, maxillary sinus wall thickness is measured at the posterolateral region where the first cut is shown when the zygoma is separated from the maxillary sinus wall, measuring the thickest part. The ethmoid sinus wall thickness is measured at the para-crista galli region around the lateral lamella, also the thickest part. The sphenoid

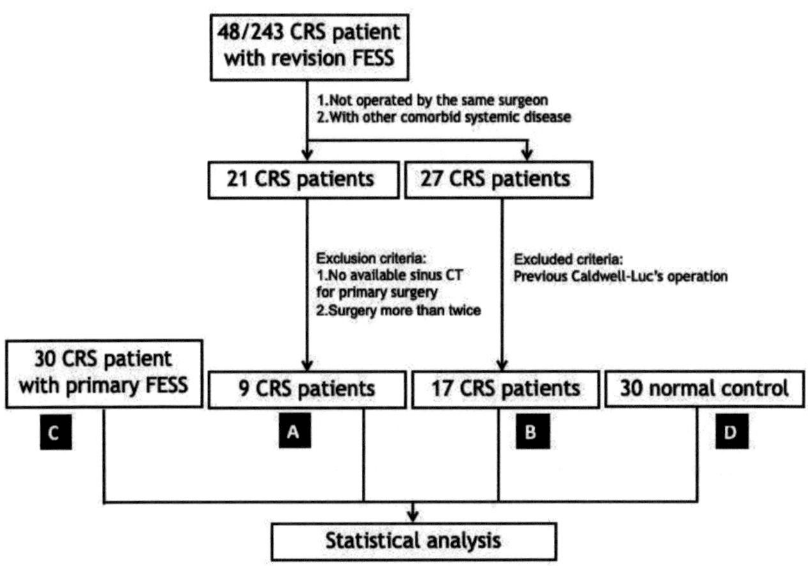

Figure 1.
Flow chart of patient selection.

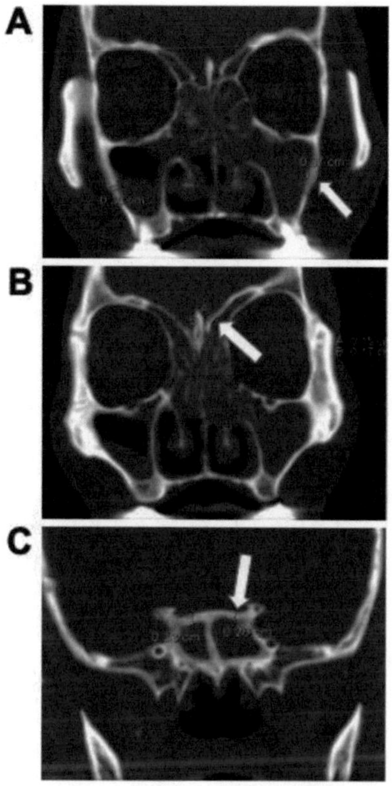

Figure 2.
Representative sinus CT scan to measure sinus wall thickness. A 61-year-old male patient with recurrent CRS and status post two times of FESS; the figure shows the preoperative sinus CT image of the first FESS. (A) Maxillary sinus wall thickness is measured at the posterolateral region. The first cut is shown when the zygoma (white arrow) is separated from the maxillary sinus wall, measuring the thickest part. (B) Ethmoid sinus wall thickness is measured at the para-crista galli region around the lateral lamella, the thickest part (white arrow). (C) The sphenoid sinus wall thickness is measured at the first cut showing the anterior clinoid, the thickest part (white arrow).

sinus wall thickness is measured at the first cut showing the anterior clinoid, the thickest part. At the lateral sphenoid wall, the carotid canal and optic nerve may introduce measurement confusion, and it is the reason why we choose the anterior clinoid level instead of the lateral sphenoid wall for wall thickness measurement where more constant sinus wall thickness could be measured. Frontal sinus wall was excluded due to its high variation of pneumatization in normal population.

We assessed gender, age, hemoglobin (Hb) levels, white blood cell (WBC) count, eosinophilic count, L-M score, bony wall thickness of maxillary/ethmoid/sphenoid sinus, and mean recurrence time of CRS. Comparisons between groups were performed by analysis of variance (ANOVA) tests for normally distributed variables and Kruskal-Wallis test for nonparametric variables, as required. Chi-square tests for categorical variables. Multiple logistic regression analysis was performed between Groups A and C against various parameters including age, gender and maxillary sinus wall thickness, LM score, Hb, and eosinophil count. Receiver-operating characteristic (ROC) curves were constructed to define cutoff value for potential refractory CRS. Linear regression was used to determine the relationship between scalar variables. All statistical analyses were performed using SPSS software. $p < 0.05$ was considered to be statistically significant.

4. Clinical features associated with the severity of CRS

4.1 Patient demographics

Group A included 8 males and 1 female (mean age, 49.1 ± 15.1 years), Group B included 11 males and 6 females (mean age, 47.8 ± 15.6 years), Group C included 23 males and 7 females (mean age, 41.9 ± 11.3 years), and Group D included 10 males and 20 females (mean age, 50 ± 14.9 years). There was no significantly difference across age (unpaired *t*-test, $p > 0.05$). The gender distribution was significantly different with obvious male preponderance in Groups A, B, and C (Kruskal-Wallis test, $p < 0.05$; **Table 1**). The information including bacteriology, eosinophilic rhinosinusitis, asthma, or ImmunoCAP Specific IgE blood test were shown in **Table 1**. The bacteriological data indicated *Staphylococcus aureus* was the major bacterial species found. The main infiltrative inflammatory cells according to pathologic slides were lymphoplasma cells and, occasionally, neutrophil infiltration. Eosinophilic rhinosinusitis was defined as average eosinophil count >10/high power field in ten randomly selected fields (X 400) under H&E staining from our previous publication [13]. Aspirin intolerance and bronchial asthma were very scarce (only one case in Groups A and C, respectively).

4.2 Hematologic examination

There was no statistically significant difference in hematologic examination results between groups (unpaired *t*-test, $p > 0.05$). The absolute peripheral eosinophil counts in Group A were significantly higher than in Group D (**Table 2**).

4.3 L-M score and sinus wall thickness

The average L-M score of Group A was 16.7 ± 8.0 and of Group C was 12.9 ± 5.1; there was no significant difference between these groups (unpaired *t*-test, $p > 0.05$, **Table 3**).

The assessments of sinus wall thickness between the independent otolaryngologists were very close. The average intraclass correlation coefficient between two assessors was 0.833 (95% confidence interval, 0.782–0.872). In terms of individual sinuses, the closest interrater agreement was found for sphenoid sinuses (0.821,

Group	N=	Age	Gender*	Bacteriology#	Eosinophilic rhinosinusitis$	Aspirin intolerance or asthma
A	9	49.1 ± 15.1	8M1F (1)&	3	1	1
B	17	47.8 ± 15.6	11M6F (3)	3	1	1
C	30	41.9 ± 11.3	23M7F (4)	2	1	0
D	30	44.7 ± 13.6	10M20F	NA	NA	NA

Group A: Revision group (same surgeon). Group B: Revision group (different surgeons). Group C: Primary FESS group. Group D: Normal control group.

$^*p < 0.05$ (Kruskal-Wallis test).

#Other than normal flora, there are Staphylococcus aureus (n = 5), MRSA (n = 1), Citrobacter koseri (n = 1), and Haemophilus influenzae (n = 1).

$Average eosinophil count >10/high power field in ten randomly selected fields (X 400) under H&E staining[13].
&Number of patient with positive ImmunoCAP test.

Table 1.
Patients' demographic data.

Group	Hematologic exam				
	Hemoglobin	WBC count (k/μl)	Eos. (%)	Peripheral eos. count (k/μl)	Sugar (g/dL)
A	14.58 ± 0.67	6333.3 ± 1494.5	4.48 ± 3.82	303.09 ± 297.48*	91.2 ± 8.3
B	14.34 ± 1.29	6119.4 ± 1781.6	2.91 ± 2.03	181.45 ± 179.31	93.1 ± 14.3
C	14.29 ± 1.53	6994.3 ± 1637.0	3.66 ± 3.03	249.48 ± 240.49	90.1 ± 9.2
D	14.00 ± 1.23	6146.7 ± 1598.4	3.50 ± 2.51	164.29 ± 204.15	96.4 ± 21.6

Group A: Revision group (same surgeon). Group B: Revision group (different surgeons). Group C: Primary FESS group. Group D: Normal control group.

**p < 0.05, compared with group D.*

Table 2.
Hematologic examination result in different groups.

Group	L-M score	Sinus wall thickness (mm)		
		Maxillary	Ethmoid	Sphenoid
A	16.7 ± 8.0	4.25 ± 1.66	1.83 ± 0.37	1.89 ± 0.66
B	12.9 ± 6.6$	2.43 ± 0.83	1.49 ± 0.28	1.49 ± 0.59
C	12.9 ± 5.1	2.06 ± 0.49¶	1.46 ± 0.24¶	1.34 ± 0.28¶
D	0.23 ± 0.43	1.97 ± 0.42¶, #	1.44 ± 0.33¶	1.39 ± 0.34¶

Group A: Revision group (same surgeon). Group B: Revision group (different surgeons). Group C: Primary FESS group. Group D: Normal control group.

¶p < 0.05, compared with group A.

#p < 0.05, compared with group B.
$With primary CT; n = 8.

Table 3.
L-M score and sinus wall thickness result in different groups.

0.932), followed by the ethmoid sinuses (0.631, 0.851) and the maxillary sinuses (0.576, 0.825). In Group A, the mean sinus wall thickness of the maxillary, ethmoid, and sphenoid sinuses were 4.25 ± 1.66 mm, 1.83 ± 0.37 mm, and 1.89 ± 0.66 mm, respectively. Group B had a mean thickness of 2.43 ± 0.83 mm, 1.49 ± 0.28 mm, and 1.49 ± 0.59 mm in the maxillary, ethmoid, and sphenoid sinuses. In Group C, the sinus wall thickness was as follows: maxillary sinus, 2.06 ± 0.49 mm; ethmoid sinus, 1.46 ± 0.24 mm; and sphenoid sinus, 1.34 ± 0.28 mm. In Group D, the measured sinus wall mean thickness of the maxillary, ethmoid, and sphenoid sinuses were 1.97 ± 0.42 mm, 1.44 ± 0.33 mm, and 1.39 ± 0.34 mm, respectively.

The sinus wall thickness of Group A was significantly higher than Groups C and D; in Group B, only the maxillary sinus wall thickness was significantly different compared to Group D (unpaired *t*-test, $p < 0.05$; **Table 3**). Multiple logistic regression analysis was performed between Groups A and C against various parameters including age, gender and maxillary sinus wall thickness, LM score, Hb, and eosinophil count. Eventually, maxillary sinus wall thickness was an independent significant factor noted ($p = 0.037$; **Table 4**).

4.4 Mean recurrence time

Average recurrence time of Group A was 28.7 ± 13.9 months. There was no significant correlation between the mean recurrence time and preoperative L-M score (**Figure 3**) or sinus wall thickness (linear regression, $p > 0.05$; **Figure 4**).

	P value	Odds ratio	95% CI
Age	0.648	1.039	0.881–1.226
Gender	0.711	0.001	0.026–8.020
Maxillary thickness	0.037	19.442	1.192–317.181
L-M score	0.958	0.994	0.800–1.235
Hb	0.648	1.400	0.330–5.951
Eosinophil count	0.827	0.999	0.989–1.009

Group A: Revision group (same surgeon). Group C: Primary FESS group.

Table 4.
Multiple logistic regression between Groups A and C.

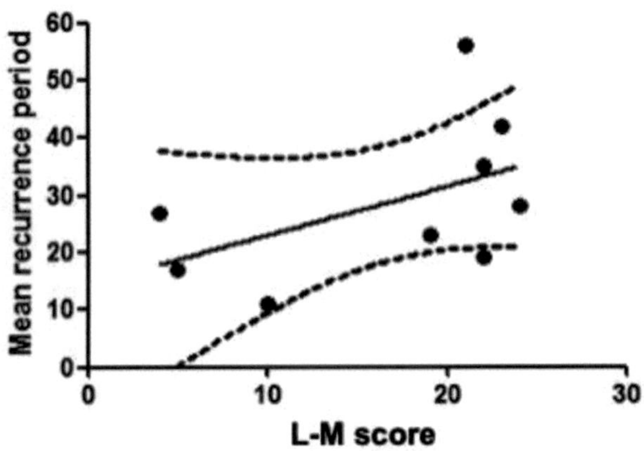

Figure 3.
Linear regression between the mean recurrence period and L-M score in Group A showed no significant relationship (p > 0.05).

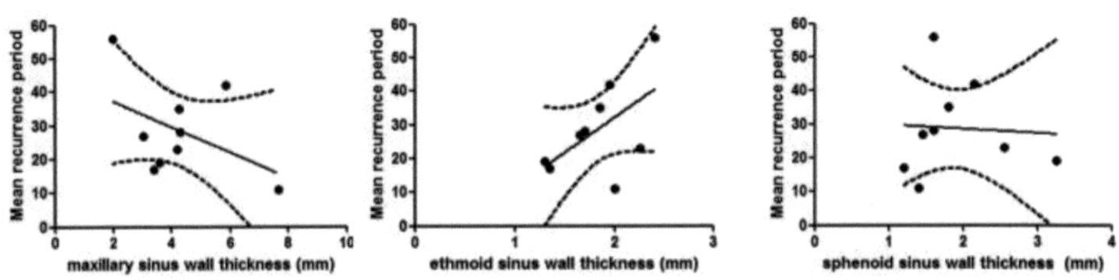

Figure 4.
Mean recurrence period showed no significant relationship compared to the maxillary, ethmoid, and sphenoid sinus wall thickness (linear regression, p > 0.05).

4.5 The cutoff values of sinus wall thickness for the prediction of recalcitrant CRS

The cutoff value of sinus wall thickness in prediction of refractory CRS who needs revision surgery differed across sinuses. The sensitivity and specificity for prediction also varied. Using 3.03 mm as a cutoff value for the maxillary sinus, the sensitivity was 88.9% and the specificity was 90%. Using 1.63 mm as cutoff value for ethmoid sinus, the sensitivity and specificity were 77.8 and 80.0%, respectively. Using 1.75 mm as a cutoff value for the sphenoid sinus, the sensitivity was 44.4% and the specificity was 80.0%.

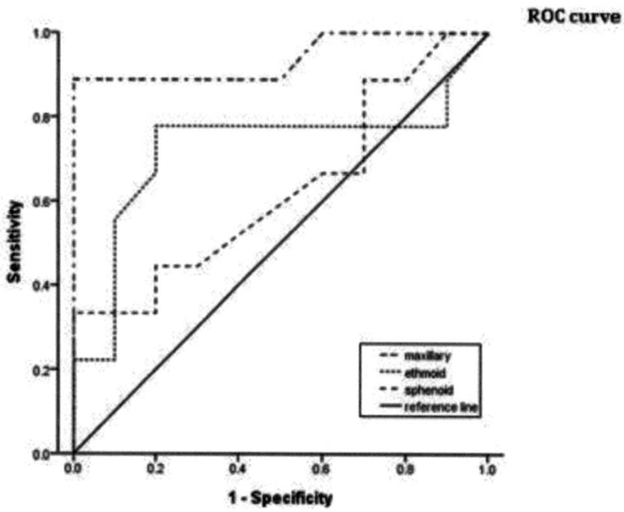

Figure 5.
ROC curve shows the cutoff values for the best sensitivity and specificity of each sinus: 3.03, 1.63, and 1.75 mm in maxillary, ethmoid, and sphenoid sinus, respectively. The ROC curve of maxillary sinus has maximal area under a curve (AUC) of 0.94.

Different sinus wall thicknesses showed areas under ROC curve (AUC) of 0.94, 0.72, and 0.63, for maxillary, ethmoid, and sphenoid sinuses, respectively. The AUC of maxillary sinus wall thickness reached statistical significance (ROC curve, $p < 0.05$; **Figure 5**).

5. Sinus wall thickness and blood eosinophilia as the indicators for revision surgeries

The success of FESS for CRS is still variable, ranging from 76 to 98% [4]. Although the exact predictive factors are still controversial, several risk factors, such as nasal polyps, allergic rhinitis, aspirin intolerance, and bacterial resistance, can result in unfavorable treatment outcomes for CRS patients. In this study, we found that the presence of thickened maxillary sinus walls of more than 3.03 mm and increased peripheral blood eosinophil count are good predictors of unfavorable outcomes from FESS. In addition to the classical L-M scoring system, a two-dimensional parameter, we suggest that these two factors may represent another three-dimensional parameter that may indicate the depth of inflammation in CRS in order to evaluate its severity.

The sinonasal organ is an expanding air-filled space that grows in a random pattern proven by using a simple computerized equation [14]. The sinus pneumatization process may be considered as using limited material ballooning to occupy the space among the eyeballs, brain, and mouth. This expanding process creates one frontal, maxillary, and sphenoid sinus cell on each side and, more importantly, the complexity of the ethmoid cell system. The bony sinus wall, which confines this sinonasal cavity, represents the boundary and most peripheral lining of this organ. If it is involved in the inflammatory process, it might be considered as one of the dimensions of the depth of disease extent, indicating a more severe form of sinonasal disease. One study showed that CRS patients had smaller maxillary sinuses than normal controls. These authors proposed that the increased bone thickness in the maxillary sinus itself might be related to the size of the sinus [15]. Accordingly, we demonstrated that maxillary sinus wall thickness is an indicator of poor surgical outcome.

The success rate of surgical outcomes for CRS patients across surgeons varies. The experience and technique of the surgeon are important factors related to the successfulness of treatment. Surgical studies contain congenital bias, that is, procedures or interventions are not executed in a uniform way; there is also a lack of patient-blinding to the surgical intervention and performance bias, which is also the case between different surgeons. Therefore, it is crucial to establish a standard surgical protocol in order to avoid the impact of the confounding effect of surgical techniques on patient outcomes. Therefore, over the past 10 years, we have made an effort to standardize surgical procedures in order to eliminate differences among surgeons. The standard eight-step FESS procedure is based on Stammberger and Kennedy's methods, which sequentially remove the obstruction of the drainage pathway anterior to posterior to reach the sphenoid sinus ostium; then, it is moved from posterior back to anterior along the identified skull base until the AEA is identified and the frontal sinus is opened. If the diseased sinuses are limited, the surgical procedure can be tailored so that the normal sinus mucosa and draining pathway are exposed and identified; this is also a way to educate beginners to understand FESS in an organized method.

In 1992, it was first suggested that chronic inflammation of the bony framework of paranasal sinuses plays a pivotal role in the pathophysiology of CRS; this hypothesis was further confirmed by subsequent animal studies [16]. Georgalas et al. proposed a global osteitis scoring scale as an indicator of revised sinus surgery [17]. Snidvongs et al. proposed that the osteitic sinus bone is a surrogate of tissue or serum eosinophilia in CRS patients [18]. Osteitis changes in the sinus bone are present in heterogeneous, irregular bone in areas of growth and destruction. Some studies have proposed that bone thickness can predict the severity of osteitis [19, 20]. Recently, sinus osteitis and subsequent bony remodeling were also suggested as a contributing factor to refractory CRS. At a microscopic level, osteitis is associated with eosinophilic inflammation and may represent a method to predict patients with P-glycoprotein overexpression by using an epithelial-to-background staining ratio; increased osteitis burden is associated with increased P-glycoprotein membranous expression in CRS [21–23]. In our study, the sinus bony walls in Group A were significantly thicker than those in Groups C and D; in Group B, only the maxillary sinus wall was significantly thicker than that of the control group. These results reflect the importance of the role of a surgeon in evaluating surgical outcomes. Our data also suggest that a posterolateral maxillary sinus wall thickness of 3.03 mm should be the cutoff value in order to predict refractory CRS.

The existence of bacterial biofilms (BBF) has also been proposed to be associated with osteitis in CRS [10]. Biofilm formation might reflect the severity, chronicity, or both of sinus infection; therefore, the release of inflammatory mediators would stimulate osteoblast activity, inducing bony remodeling and osteitis. Osteitis may further spread the pathogen either via the Haversian canal system hematogenously or from direct local invasion [24]. Intraepithelial bacteria are also found in CRS patients [25]. Considering the histology of sinus mucosa, these factors represent the depth of involvement of inflammatory process and indicate a prolonged treatment course. Although it did not reach statistical significance, maxillary sinus wall thickness is also related to shortened time to recurrence (**Figures 3** and **4**); therefore, compared to L-M scores of sinus CT, sinus wall thickness may represent greater proximity for the chronicity of CRS. At present, the mainstay of sinus surgery still focuses on restoring ventilation, yet no specific surgical method has been proven to be effective in treating osteitis associated with CRS. Instead, long-term or topical antibiotic treatment is administrated in cases of sinus osteitis and refractory sinusitis [26].

It has previously been reported that eosinophilic inflammation in the sinonasal tissues is correlated with the advanced severity of CRS and the poor outcomes associated with FESS [12]. Recent evidence has shown that eosinophilic inflammation in Caucasians CRS patients with polyps does not affect Asian to the same extent. A study from Thailand indicated a time-shifting migration of neutrophilic inflammation to eosinophilic inflammation, and a study from Korea suggested that eosinophilic inflammation might not be related to surgical outcome in Korean CRS patients [27, 28]. In our study, increased peripheral eosinophil numbers had a limited impact on surgical outcomes, suggesting that the clinical implication of eosinophilic inflammation might be different in Asian patients. Nevertheless, our study strengthens the hypothesis that increased eosinophil numbers are a poor indicator of CRS outcomes. Blood eosinophilia is induced from proliferation of eosinophil progenitor from bone marrow (myeloproliferative) or clonal expansion of peripheral eosinophil in the blood stream [29, 30]. The proposal that refractory CRS represents a local manifestation of systemic inflammatory disease is supported by our results. Our study suggested that, for those patients with obvious sinus wall thickening, more detailed preoperative consultation and laboratory tests and more aggressive postoperative medical treatment are needed.

There are several limitations of this study. First, we had small case numbers. Second, there are individual differences in the tolerance of sinusitis, as revision surgery was used as the judgment for refractory sinusitis. Despite the limitations, the knowledge gained in our study provides crucial information to guide surgical selection in CRS patients.

In summary, a variety of factors lead to refractory CRS. As a result, treatment for refractory CRS is a great challenge for ENT surgeons. Thickness of posterolateral maxillary sinus wall of more than 3.03 mm indicates possibility for revised surgery. For those CRS patients with thickened sinus wall in which we expect poor outcomes, further research is needed in order to justify the surgical procedure in such a probable systemic inflammatory disease.

6. Conclusions

In this study of subjects of chronic rhinosinusitis (CRS) undergoing functional endoscopic sinus surgery (FESS), we determined which clinical features are associated with higher possibility for revised surgery. We have developed an eight-step standard procedure to perform FESS in order to eliminate the bias of surgical technique. Sinus wall thickness and blood eosinophilia are associated with the need for revision surgery. Thickness of posterolateral sinus wall of more than 3.03 mm in maxillary sinus indicates the higher possibility for revised surgery. Also, CRS patients with thickened sinus walls were found to have poorer outcomes.

Acknowledgements

This study was supported by a grant (100-2314-B-002-044) from the Ministry of Science and Technology (MOST) of the Republic of China.

Conflict of interest

There are no financial or other relationships that could lead to a conflict of interest.

Appendices and nomenclature

CRS	Chronic rhinosinusitis
FESS	Functional endoscopic sinus surgery

Author details

Yi-Tsen Lin and Te-Huei Yeh*
Department of Otolaryngology, National Taiwan University Hospital, Taipei, Taiwan

*Address all correspondence to: tehueiyeh@ntu.edu.tw

References

[1] Jankowski R. Revisiting human nose anatomy: Phylogenic and ontogenic perspectives. The Laryngoscope. 2011;**121**(11):2461-2467. DOI: 10.1002/lary.21368

[2] Fokkens WJ, Lund VJ, Mullol J, et al. European position paper on rhinosinusitis and nasal polyps 2012. Rhinology. Supplement. 2012;**23**:1-298. DOI: 10.1055/b-0034-97635

[3] Rosenfeld RM. Clinical practice guideline on adult sinusitis. Otolaryngology and Head and Neck Surgery. 2007;**137**(3):365-377. DOI: 10.1016/j.otohns.2007.07.021

[4] Ragab SM, Lund VJ, Scadding G. Evaluation of the medical and surgical treatment of chronic rhinosinusitis: A prospective, randomised, controlled trial. The Laryngoscope. 2004;**114**(5):923-930. DOI: 10.1097/00005537-200405000-00027

[5] Georgalas C, Cornet M, Adriaensen G, et al. Evidence-based surgery for chronic rhinosinusitis with and without nasal polyps. Current Allergy and Asthma Reports. 2014;**14**(4):427. DOI: 10.1007/s11882-014-0427-7

[6] Desrosiers M. Refractory chronic rhinosinusitis: Pathophysiology and management of chronic rhinosinusitis persisting after endoscopic sinus surgery. Current Allergy and Asthma Reports. 2004;**4**(3):200-207. DOI: 10.1007/s11882-004-0027-z

[7] Lund VJ, Mackay IS. Staging in rhinosinusitis. Rhinology. 1993;**31**(4):183-184. DOI: 10.1007/978-0-387-78665-0_6567

[8] Hamilos DL. Host-microbial interactions in patients with chronic rhinosinusitis. The Journal of Allergy and Clinical Immunology. 2014;**133**(3):640-653. DOI: 10.1016/j.jaci.2013.06.049

[9] Smith TL, Mendolia-Loffredo S, Loehrl TA, et al. Predictive factors and outcomes in endoscopic sinus surgery for chronic rhinosinusitis. The Laryngoscope. 2005;**115**(12):2199-2205. DOI: 10.1097/01.mlg.0000182825.82910.80

[10] Dong D, Yulin Z, Xiao W, et al. Correlation between bacterial biofilms and osteitis in patients with chronic rhinosinusitis. The Laryngoscope. 2014;**124**(5):1071-1077. DOI: 10.1002/lary.24424

[11] Robinson JL, Griest S, James KE, et al. Impact of aspirin intolerance on outcomes of sinus surgery. The Laryngoscope. 2007;**117**(5):825-830. DOI: 10.1097/MLG.0b013e3180333121

[12] Zadeh MH, Banthia V, Anand VK, et al. Significance of eosinophilia in chronic rhinosinusitis. American Journal of Rhinology. 2002;**16**(6):313-317. DOI: 10.1177/194589240201600606

[13] Yeh TH, Hsu WC, Chen YS, et al. Decreased connexin 43 expression correlated with eosinophil infiltration in nasal polyps. American Journal of Rhinology. 2005;**19**(1):59-64. DOI: 10.1177/194589240501900110

[14] Zollikofer CP, Weissmann JD. A morphogenetic model of cranial pneumatization based on the invasive tissue hypothesis. The Anatomical Record. 2008;**291**(11):1446-1454. DOI: 10.1002/ar.20784

[15] Cho SH, Shin KS, Lee YS, et al. Impact of chronic rhinosinusitis and endoscopic sinus surgery on bone remodeling of the paranasal sinuses. American Journal of Rhinology. 2008;**22**(5):537-541. DOI: 10.2500/ajr.2008.22.3222

[16] Norlander T, Forsgren K, Kumlien J, et al. Cellular regeneration and recovery of the maxillary sinus mucosa. An experimental study in rabbits. Acta Oto-Laryngologica. Supplementum. 1992;**492**:33-37. DOI: 10.3109/00016489209136805

[17] Georgalas C, Videler W, Freling N, et al. Global osteitis scoring scale and chronic rhinosinusitis: A marker of revision surgery. Clinical Otolaryngology. 2010;**35**(6):455-461. DOI: 10.1111/j.1749-4486.2010.02218.x

[18] Snidvongs K, McLachlan R, Chin D, et al. Osteitic bone: A surrogate marker of eosinophilia in chronic rhinosinusitis. Rhinology. 2012;**50**(3):299-305. DOI: 10.4193/Rhino12.022

[19] Lee JT, Kennedy DW, Palmer JN, et al. The incidence of concurrent osteitis in patients with chronic rhinosinusitis: A clinicopathological study. American Journal of Rhinology. 2006;**20**(3):278-282

[20] Kim HY, Dhong HJ, Lee HJ, et al. Hyperostosis may affect prognosis after primary endoscopic sinus surgery for chronic rhinosinusitis. Otolaryngology and Head and Neck Surgery. 2006;**135**(1):94-99. DOI: 10.1016/j.otohns.2006.02.025

[21] Feldman RE, Lam AC, Sadow PM, et al. P-glycoprotein is a marker of tissue eosinophilia and radiographic inflammation in chronic rhinosinusitis without nasal polyps. International Forum of Allergy & Rhinology. 2013;**3**(8):684-687. DOI: 10.1002/alr.21176

[22] Bleier BS, Nocera AL, Iqbal H, et al. P-glycoprotein functions as an immunomodulator in healthy human primary nasal epithelial cells. International Forum of Allergy & Rhinology. 2013;**3**(6):433-438. DOI: 10.1002/alr.21166

[23] Gunel C, Feldman RE, Bleier BS. Osteitis is associated with P-glycoprotein overexpression in patients with chronic sinusitis without nasal polyps. American Journal of Rhinology & Allergy. 2014;**28**(2):99-102. DOI: 10.2500/ajra.2014.28.4011

[24] Perloff JR, Gannon FH, Bolger WE, et al. Bone involvement in sinusitis: An apparent pathway for the spread of disease. The Laryngoscope. 2000;**110**(12):2095-2099. DOI: 10.1097/00005537-200012000-00023

[25] Plouin-Gaudon I, Clement S, Huggler E, et al. Intracellular residency is frequently associated with recurrent *Staphylococcus aureus rhinosinusitis*. Rhinology. 2006;**44**(4):249-254

[26] Ezzat WF, Fawaz SA, Rabie H, et al. Effect of topical ofloxacin on bacterial biofilms in refractory post-sinus surgery rhino-sinusitis. European Archives of Oto-Rhino-Laryngology. 2015;**272**(9):2355-2361. DOI: 10.1007/s00405-014-3301-2

[27] Katotomichelakis M, Tantilipikorn P, Holtappels G, et al. Inflammatory patterns in upper airway disease in the same geographical area may change over time. American Journal of Rhinology & Allergy. 2013;**27**(5):354-360. DOI: 10.2500/ajra.2013.27.3922

[28] Kim SY, Park JH, Rhee CS, et al. Does eosinophilic inflammation affect the outcome of endoscopic sinus surgery in chronic rhinosinusitis in Koreans? American Journal of Rhinology & Allergy. 2013;**27**(6):e166-e169. DOI: 10.2500/ajra.2013.27.3959

[29] Simon HU, Rothenberg ME, Bochner BS, et al. Refining the definition of hypereosinophilic syndrome. The Journal of Allergy and Clinical Immunology. 2010;**126**(1):45-49. DOI: 10.1016/j.jaci.2010.03.042

[30] Valent P, Klion AD, Horny HP, et al. Contemporary consensus proposal on criteria and classification of eosinophilic disorders and related syndromes. The Journal of Allergy and Clinical Immunology. 2012;**130**(3):607, e9-612. DOI: 10.1016/j.jaci.2012.02.019

Section 3

Dental Related Sinusitis

Chapter 7

Aneurysmal Bone Cyst in Sino-nasal Region

Zeinab AlQudehy and Lena Telmesani

Abstract

Aneurysmal bone cysts (ABCs) are vascular, rapidly expanding, and locally destructive cystic lesions. It is primarily found in childhood and adolescence. They typically involve the long tubular bones. Approximately 3–6% presented in the head and neck region, with the mandible being the most common site. Involvement of the ethmoid sinuses is extremely rare with only 13 cases reported in English literatures. Here we are presenting as an example an atypical case of an adolescent male patient, which had chief complaint of right-sided nasal blockage and right eye proptosis of 6-month duration. Local examination of the face showed right eye proptosis, with bulging around the right medial canthus and lateral wall of the nose. MRI revealed multiple fluid-fluid levels of varying signal intensities on T2-weighted image suggestive of aneurysmal bone cyst. Endoscopic sinus surgery was carried out to remove the swelling and tissue specimen sent for histopathology, which confirmed the diagnosis. Patient had smooth recovery after. Throughout this chapter, we will discuss aneurysmal bone cyst from its name, origin, and histopathology. Hence, the field of interest here is sino-nasal region, thorough discussion for ABC in sino-nasal region including its clinical presentation, how to reach into diagnosis, treatment method, and finally the prognosis and recurrence.

Keywords: aneurysmal bone cyst, ethmoid sinus, pediatric, fluid-fluid level

1. Introduction

Aneurysmal bone cyst (ABC) is an uncommon cystic vascular lesion [1] that is rapidly expanding and locally destructive. It is found mostly during childhood and adolescence and is more common in females [2]. The ABC lesion typically involves the long tubular bones with approximately 3–12% presented in the head and neck region [3] and the most common site being the mandible [4]. It has been reported to arise from the sino-nasal cavity, but involvement of the ethmoid sinuses is extremely rare [3]. ABC may be found in the presence of other benign bone lesions such as non-ossifying fibroma, giant-cell granuloma, fibrous dysplasia, and fibromyxomas [1]. The rarity of this disease in the head and neck region as well as the high risk of recurrence of the lesion makes it interesting and challenging to the head and neck surgeons to deal with such pathology.

IntechOpen

2. Atypical case

A 14-year-old male patient presented with chief complaint of right-sided nasal blockage and bulging of the right eye of 6-month duration. The patient was medically free. He was in his usual state of health till 6 months prior to presentation to our clinic when he started to have nasal obstruction in the right side along with right eye proptosis. Local examination of the face showed right proptosis, with bulging around the right medial canthus and lateral wall of the nose. Nasal endoscopy by 00 rigid telescope showed poorly defined swelling in the right nasal cavity. Magnetic resonance imaging (MRI) of the nose and paranasal sinuses revealed multiple fluid-fluid levels of varying signal intensities ranging from very bright signal to a very low signal on T2-weighted image, suggestive of aneurysmal bone cyst (**Figures 1** and **2**). The patient was admitted and cleared by the ophthalmologist. Endoscopic sinus surgery

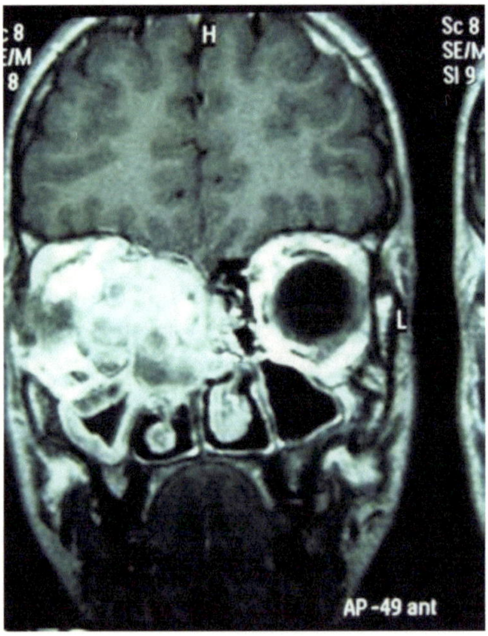

Figure 1.
MRI, coronal view showing multicystic lesion with varying intensity.

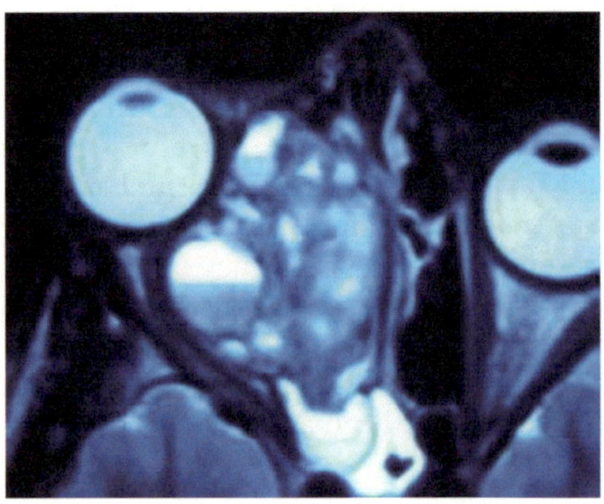

Figure 2.
MRI, axial view showing fluid-fluid levels in the lesion.

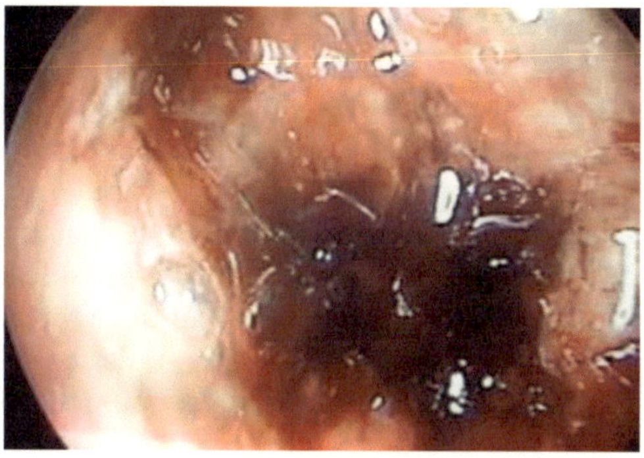

Figure 3.
Endoscopic intraoperative view of static blood inside the lesion.

was carried out to remove the nasal swelling, which showed multiple cystic swellings that were filled with blood (**Figure 3**), and tissue specimens were sent for histopathology. The histopathological specimens, on gross appearance, consist of friable hemorrhagic material that is often gritty. In en bloc resections, cyst and cortical destruction was appreciated. Microscopical results showed stroma composed of fibroblasts, multinucleate giant cells, and bone, as well as cystic spaces often filled with blood with an increased number of giant cells lining the cavity. The final histopathological diagnosis was ABC. The patient had smooth recovery postoperatively and was asymptomatic in 6 months of follow-up but unfortunately lost for subsequent follow-up after.

3. Aneurysmal bone cyst in general

3.1 History

Aneurysmal bone cysts (ABCs) were first described in 1942, by Drs. Jaffe and Lichtenstein. Typically, the described lesion was thin-walled, involving the pelvic and spine region, and they were confronted underneath large hole containing much fluid blood [5].

3.2 Characteristics of aneurysmal bone cyst

ABC is considered as uncommon benign nonneoplastic vascular lesion of the bones characterized by the presence of numerous blood-filled, usually non-epithelized cystic cavities. It is rapidly expanding and locally destructive [6].

3.3 The name of aneurysmal bone cyst

ABC is misnomer, as these lesions are neither aneurysmal in origin nor truly cystic in histopathology, with no endothelial wall. Instead, these are benign expansile lesions, within the bone, forming cavities that are filled with blood and lined by proliferative fibroblasts, giant cells, and trabecular bone [7].

3.4 Demographics of aneurysmal bone cyst

It is found mostly during childhood and adolescence, with median age of 13 years. About 90% of the ABCs lesions are found prior to age of 30. ABCs are more common in female patients, with male to female ratio of 1:1.6 [7, 8].

3.5 The origin of aneurysmal bone cyst

ABC typically originated from the long bones. It represents 1–2% of all primary tumors of the bone, occurring primarily in the metaphysis of long bones and vertebrae [8]. The ABC lesions typically involve long tubular bones. Between 3 and 12% of ABCs are found in the head and neck where they most commonly arise in the mandible or maxilla [3, 4]. Guida et al. [9] report that lesions involving the skull comprise 3–6% of all ABCs. Very few have ever been reported in the paranasal sinuses and are exceptionally rare in the pediatric population. Although they have been reported in the maxilla, mandible, cranium, orbital roof, temporal bone, and sphenoid bone, involvement of ethmoid sinuses as in our case is extremely rare [4]. Only 13 such cases of involvement of ethmoid sinuses were reported in the English literatures.

3.6 The pathogenesis of aneurysmal bone cyst

ABC's pathogenesis is obscure. Historically, it was believed that ABC resulted from increased venous pressure that is causing extravasation of cellular and blood contents into cyst-like voids in the bone [3]. More recent work showed that identification of a genetic driver—a translocation-induced upregulation of the ubiquitin-specific protease USP6 (Tre2) gene—defined at least a subset of ABCs to be a primary neoplasm [10].

3.7 Other associated bone pathologies

ABC is generally solitary and thought to arise as primary neoplasm as a result of translocation. On the other hand, ABCs may be found as secondary lesions, in the presence of other benign bone lesions such as non-ossifying fibroma, giant-cell granuloma, fibrous dysplasia, and fibromyxomas [1, 11, 12].

4. Aneurysmal bone cyst in sino-nasal region

ABC's involvement of ethmoid sinuses is extremely rare [4]. Only 13 such cases of involvement of ethmoid sinuses were reported in the English literatures. The mean age at debut in ethmoid ABCs is around 11.6 years with patient age ranging from 11 months to 20 years [3].

4.1 Clinical presentation

The diagnosis of an ABC from clinical aspect can be challenging with variable clinical presentation. Clinical presentation is highly dependent on the location of the ABC. The most common presentation of ABC in sino-nasal region relates to the presence of the expansile sockets against lamina papyracea [13]. The patient can be presented with nasal obstruction and/or facial heaviness. Epistaxis is a relatively rare presentation, since it has been reported in literatures in only two cases [3]. In the review by Hnenny et al. [14], they report that lesions affecting the skull base are more likely to present with neurological deficits including anosmia, ataxia, otalgia, facial numbness, and hearing loss.

4.2 Radiological diagnosis

Imaging studies, namely, CT scan and MRI, are essential to help with diagnosis and to plan the surgical procedure needed. ABC demonstrates the presence of expansile, lucent bony lesion surrounded by osseous remodeling and cortical thinning in CT scan [15]. In MRI images, ABC showed as multiple fluid-fluid levels of varying signal intensities. Although the fluid levels seen are nonspecific, the fact that fluid is trapped in multiple separate cavities is suggestive of ABC in both CT scan and MRI [16]. The signal characteristics are also dependent on the age of any blood products within the lesion. Other MRI features include the presence of multiple internal septations and a "soap bubble" appearance due to the presence of small cysts projected from larger cysts [13].

4.3 Definitive diagnosis

Despite all the imaging appearances suggestive of ABC, histological confirmation is essential for diagnosis. Histological evaluation of the suspected lesion is mandatory for diagnosing ABCs accurately. Ultimately, histological evaluation is key, and ABCs typically demonstrate irregular, blood-filled chambers with islands of bone and fibrous tissue [17]. In gross appearance, ABCs are spongy, hemorrhagic masses covered by a thin shell of the reactive bone. Microscopically, ABCs showed abundant red blood cells with pale brown hemosiderin that is filling cyst-like spaces and bounded by septal proliferations of fibroblasts, with mitotically active spindle cells, osteoid, calcifications, and scattered multinucleated giant cells [18]. The principal diagnostic error occurs if the histologist fails to appreciate the lining of the blood-filled spaces [2].

4.4 Treatment

The treatment of choice for ABCs is complete surgical resection, with endoscopic sinus surgery becoming the gold standard of management of aneurysmal bone cyst. Complete clearance of ABC is sometimes impossible especially at the skull base. In difficult extensive cases, further surgical procedures to debulk the lesion may be needed. Radiotherapy has been reported in cranial ABCs for refractory cases in adults. Radiotherapy has a limited success with an accepted risk of sarcomatous degeneration [9]. However, as there is a paucity of information for ethmoidal lesions particularly in children, there exists no clear consensus for radiotherapy [13].

4.5 Prognosis and recurrence

Patients needed to be followed up for quite long time with no specific adequate follow-up time reported in literatures [19]. ABCs are aggressive benign lesions with high rates of recurrence rendering its treatment uniquely challenging [20]. Recurrence can have occurred in up to 26% of cases more in jaws with most of the recurrences seem to occur within 1 year of surgical treatment [3].

5. Conclusion

Aneurysmal bone cyst is a benign, nonneoplastic lesion that presents most frequently under the age of 20 years. The metaphysis of long bones is the usual site of origin. Although the involvement of the skull is rare (2.5–6% of such cases reported in the literature), the skull vault is more often the site than the skull base. Benign ABCs are locally destructive entities which may occasionally present to otolaryngologists, since they can involve the head and neck region. ABC should be suspected, if a cystic mass in nasal cavity that is rapidly growing with fluid-fluid level in CT scan is encountered.

Acknowledgements

I acknowledge the help and support from my colleague Dr. Yasser AlNufaily, who was my assistant in conducting the endoscopic surgical removal of the case. As well as, our institution histopathology department staff who conducted an extensive review at consultant level to discuss the case and reach into the definitive diagnosis. No funding was provided to accomplish this write up for publication.

Conflict of interest

No conflict of interest.

Thanks

Thanks to our trainee resident Dr. Lina Telmsani, who helped in managing the patient's condition.

Abbreviations

ABC	aneurysmal bone cyst
ABCs	aneurysmal bone cysts

Author details

Zeinab AlQudehy[1*] and Lena Telmesani[2]

1 Dammam Medical Complex, Saudi Arabia

2 King Fahd Hospital of University, Dammam University, Saudi Arabia

*Address all correspondence to: drzeinabent@gmail.com

References

[1] Jacob G, Srugo I, Attias D, et al. Giant pediatric aneurysmal bone cysts of the occipital bone: Case report and review of the literature. Pediatric Neurology. 2011;**45**:42-44

[2] Fennessy BG, Vargas SO, Silvera MV, et al. Paediatric aneurysmal bone cysts of the head and neck. The Journal of Laryngology and Otology. 2009;**123**:635-641

[3] Girish B, Veena C, Rashmi D, Vivek CK, Rajat J. Aneurysmal bone cyst of ethmoid sinus: Uncommon manifestation of a rare case. European Journal of Radiology Extra. 2009;**70**:49-51

[4] Sanjib KU, Ashok KJ, Satyendra S, Satrughan PS, Subhash CM. Aneurysmal bone cyst of paranasal sinuses. Indian Journal of Otolaryngology and Head and Neck Surgery. 2002;**54**:305-307

[5] Hl J. Solitary unicameral bone cyst. Archives of Surgery. 1942;**44**(6):1004

[6] Jacob G et al. Giant pediatric aneurysmal bone cysts of the occipital bone: Case report and review of the literature. Pediatric Neurology. 2011;**43**(2):42-44

[7] Copley L, Dormans JP. Benign pediatric bone tumors. Evaluation and treatment. Pediatric Clinics of North America. 1996;**43**(4):949-966

[8] Leithner A et al. Aneurysmal bone cyst. A population based epidemiologic study and literature review. Clinical Orthopaedics and Related Research. 1999;(363):176-179

[9] Guida F, Rapanà A, Conti C, Cagliari E, Civelli F, Trincia G. Cranial aneurysmal bone cyst: A diagnostic problem. With a review of the literature. Child's Nervous System. 2001;**17**:297-301

[10] Ye Y et al. TRE17/USP6 oncogene translocated in aneurysmal bone cyst induces matrix metalloproteinase production via activation of NF kappaB. Oncogene. 2010;**29**(25):3619-3629

[11] Bonakdarpour A, Levy WM, Aegerter E. Primary and secondary aneurysmal bone cyst: A radiological study of 75 cases. Radiology. 1978;**126**(1):75-83. DOI: 10.1148/126.1.75

[12] Martinez V, Sissons HA. Aneurysmal bone cyst. A review of 123 cases including primary lesions and those secondary to other bone pathology. Cancer. 1988;**61**(11):2291-2304

[13] Unadkat S et al. Paediatric aneurysmal bone cyst: Not as easy as ABC. Journal of Surgical Case Reports. 2018;**2018**(2):rjy008

[14] Hnenny L et al. Giant aneurysmal bone cyst of the anterior cranial fossa and paranasal sinuses presenting in pregnancy: Case report and literature review. Journal of Neurological Surgery Reports. 2015;**76**:e216-e221

[15] Hashemi SM et al. A rare case of aneurysmal bone cyst in the paranasal sinus. Iranian Journal of Otorhinolaryngology. 2015;**27**:395-399

[16] Senol U et al. Aneurysmal bone cyst of the orbit. AJNR. American Journal of Neuroradiology. 2002;**23**:319-321

[17] Mankin HJ et al. Aneurysmal bone cyst: A review of 150 patients. Journal of Clinical Oncology. 2005;**23**:6756-6762

[18] Kumar V, Abbas AK, Aster JC. Robbins and Cotran Pathologic Basis of Disease. Philadelphia: Elsevier Saunders; 2015

[19] Bassem YS, Imad K, Jehad W, Abdulrahman E, Zoltan P. Aneurysmal bone cyst involving the skull base: A report of three cases. Skull Base Surgery. 1999;**9**:145-148

[20] Park HY et al. Current management of aneurysmal bone cysts. Current Reviews in Musculoskeletal Medicine. 2016;**9**(4):435-444

Section 4

One Airway Disease

Chapter 8

Aerosol Particles in Lungs: Theoretical Modeling of Deposition and Mucociliary Clearance

Gennady Fedorovitch

Abstract

A theoretical model of the movement of aerosols in the lungs is proposed. The model is based upon the transport equations taking into account the aerosol inertial deposition processes. Particles move along curvilinear trajectories in self-twisted vortex air flows. Deposition occurs over several cycles of inhalation and exhalation. This mechanism works for particles with a diameter greater than 1–2 microns. All particles with a diameter of 4 microns and more are captured in the respiratory tract before the terminal bronchioles. Only particles with a size of less than 2 microns can penetrate into the respiratory parts of the lungs, but the cleaning coefficient for them is close to unity. The lung cleaning model describes the limiting capabilities of the mucociliary system. The importance of taking into account the temporal characteristics of the mucociliary escalation of dust deposited in the lungs has been demonstrated. The existence of a mode of accumulation of particles in the lungs, due to a lack of cleaning time during periodic dust exposure, has been established.

Keywords: modeling, human lung, airways, swirling flow, particle deposition, distribution of aerosols, mucociliary clearance, particle transport, accumulation

1. Introduction

Rhinitis and pulmonary pathology frequently occur together. The epidemiologic, pathophysiologic, and clinical data are so compelling that the concept of "one airway, one disease" is accepted [1]. Several mechanisms have been held responsible for the interaction between the upper and lower airways (see Review [2]). A good example is the high prevalence of chronic rhinosinusitis in patients with asthma. Recent data provide ample evidence of existence of a systemic pathway between allergic rhinitis and asthma. It has been found that the severity of asthma directly correlates with the severity of sinus disease [3, 4]. Patients with chronic rhinosinusitis and asthma constitute the most severe form of unified respiratory tract disease, which is characterized by older age of the patients, greater duration of nasal symptoms, extent of sinus radiological changes, more prominent systemic inflammation markers, greater bronchial obstruction, and incidence of perennial allergic rhinitis [5].

Treating asthma with inhaled steroid therapy appears to be important in treating refractory chronic rhinosinusitis associated with asthma. In [6], the results of topical inhalation treatment of acute bacterial rhinosinusitis and standard systemic antibiotic therapy are compared. It has been found that topical inhalation therapy of acute bacterial rhinosinusitis may provide better treatment options, because systemic antibiotics can be associated with different adverse effects.

Aerosol in lungs are the task the solution of which is necessary in various areas. For example, in medical applications, aerosol therapy allows the medication to be delivered directly to those parts of the lungs where it should act.

In this chapter, we consider both deposition and clearance kinetics throughout the respiratory tract. Aerosol particles can penetrate the human lungs deep into the smallest respiratory tracts and parts of the lungs during inhalation. The effects, caused by inhaled particles, depend on the site at which they deposit within the respiratory system. Information concerning particle deposition in human lungs is of special interest because it is useful for a quantitative risk evaluation from exposure to aerosol particles. It is also vital to the effective administration of pharmaceutical aerosols by inhalation to targeted regions of the respiratory tracts. The deposition of particles in the lungs for given exposure conditions depends on parameters such as the airflow field, aerosol particle properties, breathing pattern, and geometric airway characteristics. There have been many investigations on this subject. Some recent reviews have been carried out and reported in [7–9]. In Section 3 of this chapter, we describe the aerosol inertial capture processes. Particles move along curvilinear trajectories in self-twisted vortex air flows. Deposition occurs over several cycles of inhalation and exhalation. The result is the distribution of deposition of inhaled aerosol particles in the airway generations in the respiratory tract of the lung.

Once deposited, specific clearance mechanisms will become effective, leading to a clearance of the deposited substances or a retention in different compartments of the respiratory tract. The main clearance mechanism for insoluble particles deposited in the conducting airways is via the mucociliary escalator. For the calculation of retention curves, this bronchial clearance model was applied to predicted deposition patterns for different particle sizes and breathing conditions. The importance of taking into account the temporal characteristics of the mucociliary escalation of aerosol particles deposited in the lungs has been demonstrated.

2. Model of human respiratory system

Morphometric models were initiated by E. Weibel [10] who assigned lengths and diameters to a symmetrical tracheobronchial tree (TBT) based on measurements of human airway casts. Weibel's airway tree model assumes dichotomous branching and creates a fractal structure, which is physiologically consistent in the amount of air delivered to the terminal airways and the spatial arrangement of branches within the lung. A generation is defined as all airways occurring at a specific number of bifurcations from the trachea.

The number N (i) of the branches of the ith generation and the diameter D (i) are given by the formulas

$$N(i) = 2^{i}\ ;\ D(i) = D(0) * 2^{-i/3} \tag{1}$$

The airway diameter decreases distally, but because of the increasing number of tubes, the total cross section increases and the air velocity decreases. The law of change of air velocity follows from the requirement of conservation airflow before and after dividing branches of TBT:

$$V(i) = V(0) * 2^{-i/3} \tag{2}$$

The trachea (0th generation) has $D(0) = 1.44$ cm and $V(0) = 290$ cm/s. The branches of the 18th generation correspond to terminal bronchioles. The radius $R(i) = D(i)/2$, and length $L(i)$ of each branch is assumed to be equal to three times the diameter.

In the adopted model, the time tp for the passage of the air channel is the same for all generations:

$$t_p = L(i)/V(i) = 3 * D(i)/V(i) = 3 * D(0)/V(0) \approx 0.015 \text{ sec}. \tag{3}$$

We can compare this time with the characteristic inhalation time $t_{in} = 1.25$ s (we assume that the breathing frequency is 12 1/min, and for each period, there are four identical phase durations: inhale, pause, exhale, and pause). The ratio $t_{in}/t_p \approx 100$ can be considered as the possible number of TBT generations that air could pass during inhalation. As was to be expected, this number is significantly greater than the total number of generations (≈ 25) of TBT. The passage of the airways to the level of the alveoli takes no more than 10% of the total inhalation time.

2.1 Air flow characteristics

An important dimensionless quantity in air mechanics is the Reynolds number (Re). It is used in the scaling of similar but different sized flow situations [11]. The value of Re is the ratio of inertial forces to viscous forces within an air which is subjected to relative internal movement due to different air velocities, which is known as a boundary layer in the case of a bounding surface such as the interior of an airway. In the air channel of TBT, the Reynolds number can be defined as

$$Re(i) = V(i) * R(i)/\nu \tag{4}$$

where ν is the air kinematic viscosity. The Reynolds number is important for different situations where a fluid is in relative motion to a surface. Matching the Reynolds numbers in different airways is sufficient to guarantee similitude of airflows. **Table 1** shows the Reynolds numbers characterizing the air flow in the respiratory tract.

It can be seen that in almost all branches of the TBT, the flow is laminar, however with $Re > 1$.

The behavior of particles suspended in an air flow is characterized [11] by Stokes number (Stk). It is defined as the ratio of the characteristic time of an aerosol particle to a characteristic time of the flow. In the air channel of TBT, the Stokes number can be defined as

$$Stk = (1/18) * \left(\rho_p/\rho_a\right) * \left(d_p{}^2/\nu\right) * [V(i)/R(i)] \tag{5}$$

i=	0	2	4	6	8	10	12	14	16	18	20
Re =	1392.0	552.4	219.2	87.0	34.5	13.7	5.4	2.2	0.9	0.3	0.1

Table 1.
Reynolds numbers in the branches of the TBT.

d_p, μm	1	2	4	6	10	20	40
Stk =	0.0015	0.0060	0.024	0.054	0.149	0.60	2.39

Table 2.
Stokes numbers for particles of different diameters.

where ρ_p and ρ_a are the particle and air densities and d_p is the particle diameter. Value $R(i)/V(i)$ is the characteristic time of the flow. A particle with a low Stokes number follows fluid streamlines, while a particle with a large Stokes number is dominated by its inertia and continues along its initial trajectory. For $Stk \gg 1$, particles will detach from a flow especially where the flow decelerates abruptly. For $Stk \ll 1$, particles follow fluid streamlines closely.

In the accepted TBT model, the ratio of air velocity to diameter is the same for all generations; therefore, the Stokes number is the same in all branches, and it changes depending on the particle diameter. The corresponding results are shown in **Table 2**.

It can be seen that particles with a diameter of up to 10 μm ($Stk \ll 1$) are involved in the movement of air. Only particles with a large diameter can "break away" from the flow and, for example, settle onto the wall directly due to the inertial mechanism.

2.2 Mucociliary escalator

The kinetics of mechanical particle transport from the TBT via the mucociliary escalator to the larynx cannot be measured directly. Average tracheal mucus velocities in healthy nonsmokers, as measured by noninvasive radiological techniques, ranged from 4 to 6 mm/min consequently; both ICRP [12] and NCRP [13] committees adopted a value of 5.5 mm/min. Because of the very limited experimental data on mucus clearance velocities in human bronchial airways, mucus velocity in other bronchial airways has to be calculated, using assumptions about TBT morphology and properties of the mucus flow in these airways. The law of change of mucus velocity $U(i)$ follows from the requirement of conservation flows before and after dividing branches of TBT:

$$2 * \pi * D(i) * U(i) = \pi * D(i-1) * U(i-1) \tag{6}$$

The diameter of each airway is determined by (1). So, we have

$$U(i) = U(0) * 2 - 2i/3 \tag{7}$$

This model uses an empirically derived expression for mucociliary transport rates in TBT.

For the calculation of retention characteristics, this bronchial clearance model was applied to predicted deposition patterns for different particle sizes and breathing conditions.

3. Inertial capture

Inertial capture of aerosol particles from air flow is illustrated by **Figure 1**.

Particles entering the channel near the center fly through it during the time of the $t_p \approx 0.015$ sec (see above Section 2.1.). Particles entering the channel near the

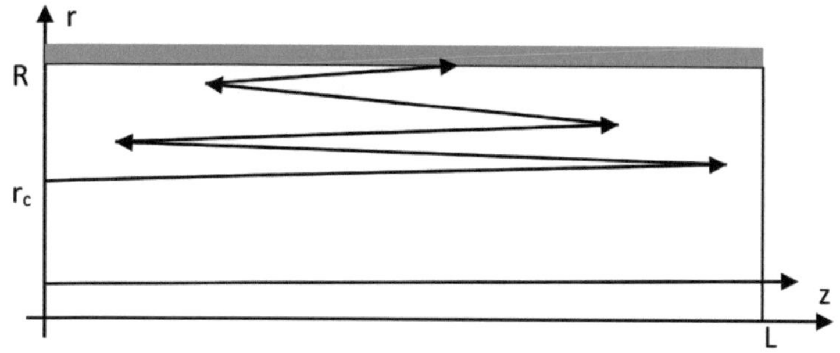

Figure 1.
Trajectories of particles entering the air flow in a straight pipe with round cross section at distances r_c from the center. A cylindrical coordinate system (r,z) is used. The airway radius is R; length is L.

wall move more slowly due to the effect of deceleration of the air flow in the boundary layer. During inhalation, they may not reach the end of the channel. They turn back during exhalation.

An important circumstance is the air swirling flow at the point of bifurcation of the branches of TBT [7]. Numerical studies on the bifurcation flow of lung models consistently identified different types of secondary flow pattern such as swirl-flow pattern or double vortex, also known as Dean flow. At inspiration, the rate of swirling flow at the inlet to the branch of TBT is 20–25% of the axial velocity.

In such a flow, the centrifugal force shifts the particles to the wall. Here, the particle is additionally inhibited. After several cycles of "inhale-exhale," the particle will deposit on the wall. The capture of particles in some branch of the TBT occurs if the transit time of this branch is longer than the inhalation time tin$\approx$ 1.25 s (see Section 1). The transit time increases with increasing distance from the channel axis. The particles that fly into the airway at a distance r > rc from axis are captured. This condition determines the probability P (i) of particle capture in the ith branch of the TBT:

$$P(i) = \left(\pi R^2 - \pi r_c{}^2\right)/\pi R^2 = 1 - r_c{}^2/R^2 \qquad (8)$$

This mechanism is the most effective even for small aerosol particles.

3.1 Air flow characteristics

There are numerous research studies focusing on airflow in the respiratory system (see Review [14]). The results of these studies provide an almost complete picture of the airflow in the lungs. It is easy to recognize the "classical" flow patterns in smooth cylindrical tubes (see [11]).

The axial velocity distribution at the entrance can be considered uniform. Further downstream, a Prandtl boundary layer forms along the walls. Its thickness is gradually increasing. In sufficiently long pipes at a distance Le from the entrance, the boundary layer fills the entire cross section. It establishes a Poiseuille flow with a parabolic distribution of the axial velocity along the radius r. The steady-state flow does not depend on the velocity distribution at the inlet. The distance at which the Poiseuille flow is formed is called the input length L_e. For L_e we have

$$L_e \approx 0.1 * D * R_e \qquad (9)$$

For a small (compared to the channel radius) thickness of the boundary layer, the axial air velocity V_z is described by the relation (Blasius solution):

$$V_z = V_{in} * f\ (\zeta) \tag{10}$$

where V_{in} is the velocity far from the wall, which can be equated to the velocity at the entrance to the channel, and ζ is the self-similar variable:

$$\zeta = (R - r) * [V_{in}/z\,\nu]^{1/2} \tag{11}$$

The function f (ζ) is the result of a numerical solution of the continuity and Navier–Stokes equations after the transition to the self-similar variable ζ. The function f (ζ) initially grows linearly with increasing ζ and then approaches to 1. The scale of change is $\zeta_0 \approx 3$.

The swirling of the air flows was found in the numerical simulation of currents in the TBT channels [15, 16]. The distribution of the azimuthal velocity V_φ along the radius in the cross section of the channel is well interpolated by the function

$$V_\varphi = S * V_{in} * (r/R) * (1 - r/R) \tag{12}$$

This function describes the real decrease in azimuthal velocity as it approaches the axis and the channel wall. The intensity of the vortex (swirl number) S is defined as the ratio of the average over the cross-sectional azimuthal velocity V_φ to axial velocity V_z. At the entrance to the air channel of the TBD, the value of $S = S0 \approx 0.15–0.25$ [15], and then S (z) decreases exponentially. The characteristic decay distance is close to the input length L_e [17].

3.2 Model of the capture of aerosol particles

This data is sufficient to make an estimate of the probability of the capture in the ith branch of the TBT. The motion of aerosol particles along the z axis is determined by the speed [Eq. (10)]. In the radial direction, the aerosol particle moves under the action of centrifugal force:

$$3 * \pi * d_p * \rho_a * \nu * (dr/dt) = m * {V_\varphi}^2/r \tag{13}$$

Time does not explicitly enter into Eqs. (10) and (13). They define (r, z) trajectory. In dimensionless variables $x = z/R$ and $y = r/R$, this trajectory is described by the formula

$$y = y_1/\left\{y_1 + (1 - y_1) * \exp.\left[-(2/3) * \Gamma^2 * Stk * \zeta_o * x^{3/2}/Re^{1/2}\right]\right\} \tag{14}$$

Here, $y_1 = r_1/R$ is the dimensionless radius of the particle entrance. The full trajectory will be obtained after twisting (r, z) trajectories around the axis of the channel in accordance with the rotation of the particles with the azimuthal velocity V_φ along with the flow.

From Eq. (14), it follows that if $Re \gg 1$ (initial generation of TBT) and/or $Stk \ll 1$ (small particle size), then $y \approx y_1$ all the way. In this instance, the particles do not shift to the wall. The shift is noticeable in those air channels where

$$\lambda = (2/3) * \Gamma^2 * Stk * \zeta_o * {x_c}^{3/2}/Re^{1/2} > 1 \tag{15}$$

Even if $\lambda \ll 1$, always $y < 1$, that is, direct deposition of particles due to their centrifugal demolition to the channel walls does not occur. However, the removal of particles into the zone of slow near-wall flow can significantly increase the time of flight of the particle through the channel. The definition of the transit time can be obtained, for example, by integrating the equation of motion for x ($\tau = t^*V_{in}/R$). The estimate of the channel transit time τ_c, taking into account the removal of a particle into the zone of a slow near-wall flow, has the form:

$$\tau_c = \{\lambda + [\exp(\lambda) - 1] * y_1/(1 - y_1)\}/\mathrm{Stk} * \Gamma^2 \quad (16)$$

As λ increases to large values, the time span τc grows exponentially and can reach values greater than the inspiratory time. This can be considered the effect of trapping a particle in the corresponding channel. According to Eq. (16), the value of τ_c is different for particles entering the channel at different distances y_1 from the center of the channel. Only particles are captured that enter the channel at distances greater than that determined from the equation

$$y_1/(1 - y_1) = [\Gamma^2 * \mathrm{Stk} * \tau_{in} - \lambda]/[\exp(\lambda) - 1] \quad (17)$$

The dimensionless inspiratory time τ_{in} is defined in Section 2.1; it is ≈ 250.

The right-hand side of Eq. (17) varies with the generation number and with the characteristics (mass and size) of aerosol particles. Changes in the entrance radius of the capture of particles at the channel entrance lead to changes (according to Eq. (8)) of the probability of their settling in the ith generation.

3.3 Results

The results of the calculation of the probability of the capture of particles of different diameters in the generation of the respiratory tract TBT are presented in **Figure 2**.

It can be seen that the air cleaning mechanism due to the capture of aerosols in the airways is quite effective even for particles with a diameter of 1–2 μm. Particles with a diameter of 4 μm and more are almost completely captured in channels with a generation number < 19, that is, to respiratory branches of TBT. Particles of large diameters (>10 μm) are captured in the upper respiratory tract, that is, the

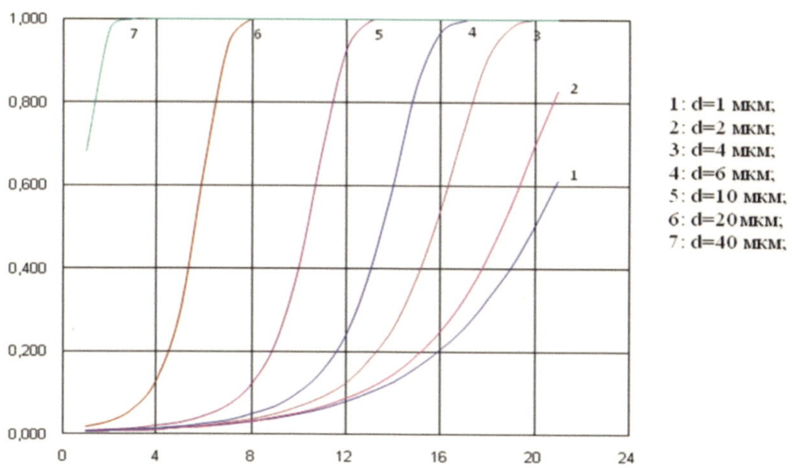

Figure 2.
Dependence of the probability P of the capture of a particle (ordinates) with diameter d in the respiratory tracts of the ith generation (abscissa axis) of TBT.

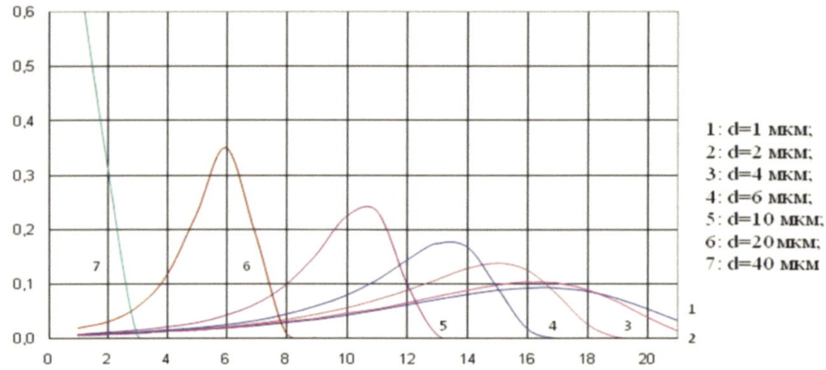

Figure 3.
The distribution of trapped particles of different diameters d by the numbers of generation of TBT.

trachea, the zonal extrapulmonary bronchi, and the intrapulmonary subsegmental bronchi.

The probability of capture (formula Eq.(8)) determines the proportion of captured particles from the total number of particles entering the channel. It is possible to determine the probability Pa (i) of the particles reaching the ith generation:

$$Pa(i) = \prod_{k=0}^{k=i-1} [1 - P(k)] \tag{18}$$

The probability of reaching the deep parts of the lungs is almost zero for particles with sizes larger than 10 microns. Particles with sizes of 4–6 microns can penetrate into the lungs only up to the terminal bronchioles. Only particles with a size of less than 2 microns can penetrate into the respiratory branches of the TBT, but the cleaning coefficient for them is close to 1. These data also indicate a high efficiency of the capture of particles as a mechanism for cleaning air from aerosols.

Finally, we present data on the probability of trapping particles in the airway of the TBT. Denoting this value as P_c (i), we can calculate it using the obvious formula

$$P_c(i) = P_a(i) * P(i) \tag{19}$$

The results of the calculation of P_c (i) are shown in **Figure 3**.

The latter result gives a clear picture of the areas of the lungs in which the capture of aerosol particles of different diameters occurs. It is seen that even the smallest particles are mainly trapped in the bronchioles to the respiratory part. Large particles (with a diameter of 6 microns and more) do not penetrate into the terminal bronchioles at all.

4. Model of mucociliary clearance of the lungs

As a rule, the modification of the model of E. Weibel leads to more realistic conclusions about the work of the lungs. In addition, it allows us to describe a number of effects that are impossible in the "classical" TBT model. There are, however, negative aspects of such a modification. Asymmetric statistical models are analyzed only by numerical methods. At the same time, however, the visibility of the results and the possibility of generalization the conclusions are lost. Therefore, for the initial estimates, it is advisable to limit ourselves to the simpler initial morphometric model of E. Weibel.

4.1 Formulation of the problem

We introduce adequate variables to describe the dynamics of mucociliary cleaning of the lungs. We will describe the flow j (z, t) of the mucociliary escalation by the product of the velocity U(z) and the density n (z, t). The latter is the number of aerosol particles per unit length of the corresponding generation of TBT. Here and later, t is time, and z is the coordinate along the TBT generations. It is counted from the larynx. Here, the advantage of considering generations instead of TBT branches is used explicitly. Generation is the entire set of TBT branches with the same division number. If you follow the flow of particles along the branches of the TBT, it will have gaps (vary approximately twice) at the points of division. If the flow is attributed to generation, it will be continuous. The continuity equation will be

$$\frac{\partial n}{\partial t} - \frac{\partial Un}{\partial z} = q(x, t) \tag{20}$$

Here, q (z, t) denotes the density of aerosol deposition on the inner surface of the TBT (per unit generation length and per unit time). Since precipitation occurs faster (in a few breath-exhalation cycles) than cleaning the lungs, sedimentation density can be factorized:

$$q(z, t) = Q(z) * H(t) \tag{21}$$

Here, the function H (t) describes the temporal dependence of the entry of aerosol particles into the lungs, and Q (z) is the distribution of the trapped particles along the TBT generations. The latter function is directly related to the probability of capture P_i found in Section 3. To determine the relationship, let us establish the correspondence of the z coordinate to the generation number i. Choosing the origin (z = 0) at the beginning of the trachea, we get that the end of the ith generation corresponds to the coordinate

$$z = z_i \equiv \sum_{k=0}^{k=i} l_k \tag{22}$$

Here, l_k is the length of the kth generation. In the model of E. Weibel, it changes with the number k as well as the diameter: $l_k = l_0 {*} 2^{-k/3}$. The geometric progression (Eq. (22)) is summed. For z_i we have

$$z_i = l_0 * \frac{1 - 2^{-(i+1)/3}}{1 - 2^{-1/3}} = Z * \left(1 - 2^{-\frac{i+1}{3}}\right) \tag{23}$$

Here, $Z = l_0 / (1{-}2^{-1/3}) \approx 29.1$ cm is the total length of the TBT generations. The distribution of trapped particles Q (z) can be determined through the air exchange rate in the lungs W and the concentration of particles R in inhaled air:

$$Q(z) = W * R * P_i / l_i \tag{24}$$

We can express the mucociliary velocity U in terms of the z coordinate along the TBT generations:

$$U(z) = U_0 * (1 - z/Z)^2 \tag{25}$$

where $U0 \approx 2.4 * 10^{-2}$ cm/s is the velocity at the entrance to the TBT (near the larynx). With such values of the scale of length and velocity, the time scale is $T = Z/U0 \approx 1.2*10^3$ sec = 0.337 hour. The relation (Eq. (25)) is valid only at the bifurcation points, but in the future, it is also advisable to use it at intermediate values of z.

Instead of the density n (z, t), we introduce a new variable—the stream j (z, t) = n (z, t) * U (z), and instead of the z coordinate, a new variable

$$\vartheta(x) = \int_0^x dx/U(x) \tag{26}$$

The meaning of this variable is the time required for the escalation of particles from depth z to the TBT. For the dependence U (z) given by formula (Eq. (25)), we obtain

$$\frac{\vartheta}{T} = \frac{z/Z}{1 - z/Z}; \frac{z}{Z} = \frac{\vartheta/T}{1 + \vartheta/T} \tag{27}$$

From Eq. (20) we obtain the equation for the flow:

$$\frac{\partial j}{\partial t} - \frac{\partial j}{\partial \vartheta} = q(\vartheta, t) * U(\vartheta) \tag{28}$$

Its solution for the natural boundary conditions ($j \to 0$ as $\vartheta \to \infty$ or $t \to -\infty$) has the form:

$$j(\vartheta, t) = \int_0^\infty q(\vartheta + u, t - u) * U(\vartheta + u) * du \tag{29}$$

Solution (Eq. (29)) of the problem of the dynamics of mucociliary clearance of the lungs allows us to estimate the parameters of escalation in several practically important cases.

4.2. Examples of solutions

Let us consider, for example, the dynamics of excretion of particles inhaled in a short time T0. In this case, the time dependence of the settling of particles can be chosen in the form $H(t) = T_0 * \delta(t)$, where δ (t) is the Dirac impulse delta function.

The presence of the delta function allows us to determine the integral (29) and record the outflow of TBT (with z = 0) of the flow of settled particles in the form

$$j(z = 0, t) = T_0 WR[U(z) * P_i/l_i]_{z = z(t)} \tag{30}$$

The content of square brackets in this ratio is taken for z, which varies with time according to Eq. (27). The results of calculations of the time dependence of the removal of particles of different diameters are shown in **Figure 4**.

As was to be expected, particles of large diameters (10–20 μm), which are captured in proximal sections of the TBT (generation with number i = 6–11), are removed in the first hours (5–9 hours). This can be explained by the high rate of mucociliary escalation ($U = 10^{-3}$–10^{-4} cm/s). The maximum is clearly visible in the time dependence of the flow. Small particles (d = 1–4 μm) are removed much more slowly (1 day or more), and the time dependence of the flux decreases monotonously.

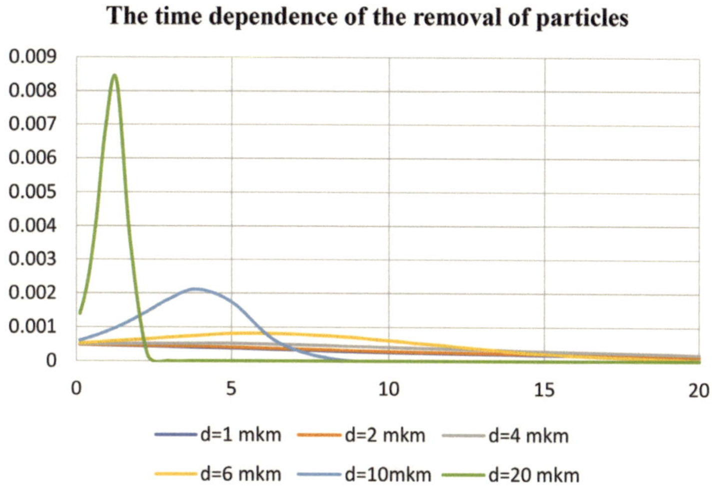

Figure 4.
Dependence on time t (hour) of the particle flux at the exit of TBT.

Integration over time of the effluent (30) gives us

$$\int_0^{\infty} j(o,t)dt = T_0 WR \int_0^{Z} (P_i/l_i)dz = > (dz = l_i di) = > T_0 WR \sum P_i = T_0 W \quad (31)$$

The last equality indicates the preservation of the number of aerosol particles: the total number of particles released (left side of Eq. (31)) is equal to the number of inhalation particles (right side of Eq. (31)).

We get other results in the case of prolonged (many hours) inhalation of dusty air. This situation is realized in the case of industrial dust exposure, which continues during the work shift. We assume that such an effect begins at $t = 0$ and stops at $t = t0 = 8$ hours. In this case, the function H (t) in the relation (Eq. (21)) can be given by the formula

$$H(t) = \eta(t) * \eta(t_0 - t) \quad (32)$$

Here, η (t) is the unit Dirac function, which is zero for negative values of the argument and one for positive.

In this case, the solution (Eq. (29)) of Eq. (28) can be written as

$$j(\vartheta, t) = \left\{ \begin{array}{cc} 0 & \text{if } t < 0 \\ \int_{\vartheta}^{\vartheta+t} Q(\vartheta')v(\vartheta')d\vartheta' & \text{if } t_0 > t > 0 \\ \int_{\vartheta+t-t_0}^{\vartheta+t} Q(\vartheta')v(\vartheta')d\vartheta' & \text{if } t > t_0 \end{array} \right\} \quad (33)$$

Interesting is the observed value of the flow of precipitated particles at the exit from the TBT, with $\vartheta = 0$. If we return from the variable ϑ to the coordinate z, we get

$$j(0, t > 0) = \int_{z_1}^{z_2} Q(z')dz' \quad (34)$$

where

z_2 (t) $= U_0 * t/[1 + U_0 * t/Z]$; z_1 (t) $= 0$ for $t < t_0$ and z_1 (t) $= z_2$ $(t - t_0)$ for $t > t_0$.

Formula (34) clearly demonstrates where the deposited particles are drawn from at a certain point in time.

Dependences on time t are depicted graphically in **Figure 5**. Along the abscissa, the time (in hours) after the start of inhalation of aerosol particles (10 μm in diameter) is plotted. Inhalation is assumed to occur over a period of time from t = 0 to t_0 = 8 hours. The boundaries z_1 and z_2 of the integration range are represented by the corresponding curves. The sedimentation density distribution of particles along the z coordinate (the integrand function Q (z) in the formula (Eq. (34)) is shown in the same graph. It can be seen that in the first hours after the start of inhalation, particles are removed from the TBT sections that are at a distance from the beginning to ≈ 0.8 * Z. A small part of the aerosol particles is captured here. Over time, the length of the cleaning section increases. After 5 hours, the removal of particles from a depth of ≈ 0.94 * Z begins. From here, a significant part of the trapped aerosol particles is removed. The maximum elimination occurs at t ≈ 10 hours after the start. After this, the boundaries of the dust removal area are shifted further into TBT, where relatively little dust accumulates. By 15–20 hours after the start of inhalation (7–12 hours after the end), almost all captured particles are removed from TBT.

Thus, breaks lasting 7-12 hours eliminate the risk of accumulation of aerosol particles with a diameter of 10 mkm in the lungs. It is assumed, of course, that the mass of the trapped aerosol particles is not too large, so that its removal does not exceed the mass transfer capabilities during mucociliary escalation.

Cleaning the lungs from smaller dust particles occurs differently. The most probable capture depth is ≈ 0.98 * Z for particles with g = 4 μm. In these generations of TBT, the rate of mucociliary escalation is 10 times less than in the trachea. Cleaning time is much longer.

The results of direct calculations of the flow at the TBT outlet confirm these conclusions (see **Figure 6**).

It is seen that particles with d = 20 μm practically do not stay in the lungs; they come out of TBT as they arrive, of course, if the mass of trapped particles does not exceed the mass transfer capacity during mucociliary escalation. Particles with d < 4 μm are deposited in the deep sections of TBT. They do not have time to get out of the lungs during the break. Their share exceeds 30%. This indicates the possibility of accumulation in the lungs of trapped particles of small diameter. For almost

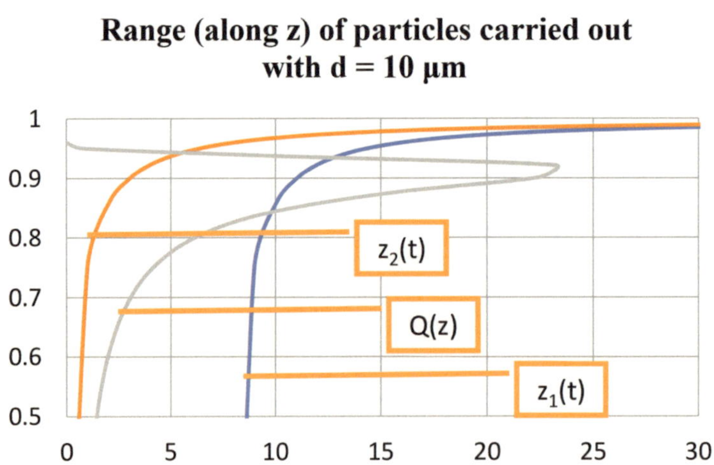

Figure 5.
The dependence on time t (hour) of the boundaries of removal from the TBT trapped particles with a diameter of 10 mkm.

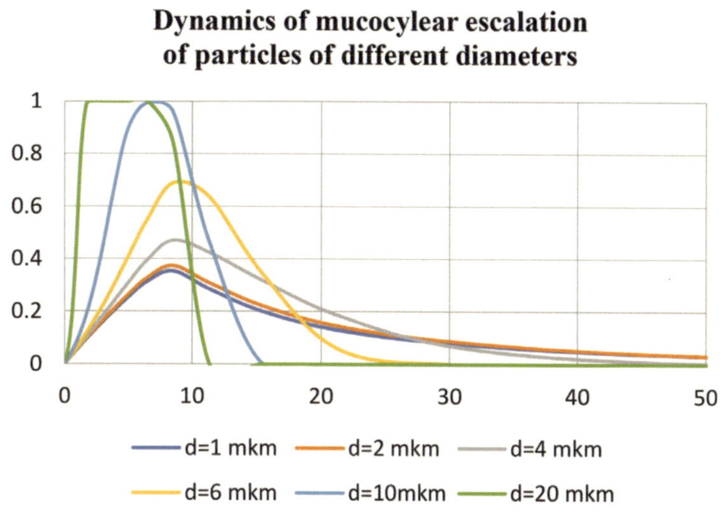

Figure 6.
The time dependence of the elimination of aerosol particles trapped in 8 hours of work.

complete removal of such particles, it is necessary not less than 2 days. More time is needed to remove smaller particles.

The fact of accumulation of small particles during periodic inhalation of dusty air (during working hours), alternating with periods of rest when mucociliary clearance of the lungs occurs, raises the question of the average number of particles characterizing the result of such accumulation. Using solution (Eq. (33)) of Eq. (20), which describes the dynamics of mucociliary cleaning of the lungs, we can determine the density n (z, t) of the captured particles n(z, t) = j (z, t) / U (z). And after integrating by TBT generation, we have the total amount of N (t) particles in the lungs:

$$\mathrm{N(t)} = \int_0^Z \mathrm{dz}\frac{\mathrm{j(z,t)}}{\mathrm{U(z)}} = \int_0^\infty d\vartheta j(\vartheta,\mathrm{t}) = \int_0^\infty d\vartheta \int_0^\infty d\tau q(\vartheta+\tau,\mathrm{t}-\tau)\mathrm{v}(\vartheta+\tau) \qquad (35)$$

Obvious substitutions of order and integration variables simplify this expression to the form:

$$\mathrm{N(t)} = \int_0^\infty d\vartheta U(\vartheta)\mathrm{Q}(\vartheta)\int_0^\vartheta d\tau H(\mathrm{t}-\tau) \qquad (36)$$

Now, the time dependence of the capture of particles H (t) is a sequence of rectangular pulses of the form (Eq. (32)), duration t0 (working time), and periodicity t_1 (1 day). A rigorous computation of the double integral (Eq. (36)) is possible, but not interesting. It is clear that this is a certain function of time, which varies with the period of the day around a certain mean value <N>. It can be estimated quite accurately. Indeed, the calculation of the average < N > in time from N (t) reduces to replacing in the integral H (t-τ) by <H (t-τ)>. The last value does not depend on τ; therefore, from Eq. (36) we can get

$$<N> = <H> * \int_0^\infty d\vartheta v(\vartheta)\mathrm{Q}(\vartheta)\vartheta - <H> * \int_0^X \mathrm{dxQ(x)}\vartheta(\mathrm{x}) \qquad (37)$$

As in formulas (Eq. (26–27)), the meaning of the variable ϑ (z) is the time required for the escalation of particles from depth z to the beginning of the TBT.

d, mkm	1	2	4	6	10	20
$<\vartheta>$,hours	27.7	23.7	12.3	7.4	3.6	1.1

Table 3.
The average exit time for particles of different diameters.

The same technique that was used in the transition in formula (Eq. (21)) from the integral to the sum over the generation numbers leads to the expression

$$<N> = <H> * W * R * <\vartheta> \tag{38}$$

Here, the average exit time $< \vartheta >$ is determined by the probability distribution of the capture of particles of the corresponding diameter:

$$<\vartheta> = \sum P_i * \vartheta_i \tag{39}$$

The relation (Eq. (38)) is quite clearly interpreted: the average number of aerosol particles in the lungs is equal to their number in the volume of air, which is determined by pulmonary air exchange over the average time of exiting $<\vartheta>$.

The obtained values of the average time of exit are in complete agreement with the results on the time dependence of the output stream for various inhalation regimes given above. The average exit time for particles of different diameters is given in **Table 3**.

5. Conclusions

We investigated the deposition, retention, and clearance of inhaled aerosol particles in the lungs. Each of these processes is intensively investigated in numerous papers. As a rule, for their analysis, complex computer simulation of air and hydrodynamic flows in the branches of TBT is used.

The phenomenological model we have constructed is a simplified picture of real processes. It is used to study the key aspects of aerosol behavior in the lungs. This is a self-consistent and closed set of assumptions about the process, reflecting the basic, though not all, properties of a real phenomenon. Simulation is a research method with several goals:

- Structuring existing knowledge, giving it a certain shape, turning a data set into some information design

- The use of already accumulated information to determine the priority directions of its detailed elaboration, ranking of new information

The model reflects the unity of the main functional structures and, at the same time, the specifics of the processes occurring in them. Despite the descriptive nature of the proposed modeling, its meaning is that it gives the plot accuracy and compositional clarity, which are not inherent in real objects of modeling.

Conflict of interest

The author does not have a conflict of interest.

Author details

Gennady Fedorovitch
NTM-Defense, Moscow, Russia

*Address all correspondence to: fedorgv@gmail.com

References

[1] Bousquet J, Khaltaev N, Cruz AA, et al. Allergic rhinitis and its impact on asthma (ARIA). Allergy. 2008;**63**: 8-160

[2] Malaty J. Medical management of chronic rhinosinusitis in adults. Sinusitis. 2016;**1**(1):76-87

[3] Braunstahl GJ, Overbeek SE, Fokkens WJ, et al. Segmental bronchoprovocation in allergic rhinitis patients affects mast cell and basophil numbers in nasal and bronchial mucosa. American Journal of Respiratory and Critical Care Medicine. 2001;**164**: 858-865

[4] Beeh KM, Beier J, Kornmann O, et al. A single nasal allergen challenge increases induced sputum inflammatory markers in non-asthmatic subjects with seasonal allergic rhinitis: Correlation with plasma interleukin-5. Clinical and Experimental Allergy. 2003;**33**:475-482

[5] Chen YT, Chien CY, Tai SY, et al. Asthma associated with chronic rhinosinusitis: A population-based study. International Forum of Allergy & Rhinology. 2016;**6**(12):1284-1293

[6] Pshennikov DS, Angotoeva IB. The prospects for inhalation therapy of rhinosinusitis. Eruditio Juvenium. (http://paper.researchbib.com/view/paper/136231). 2017;**5**(2):277-282

[7] Gemci T, Ponyavin V, Chen Y, Chen H, Collins R. Computational model of airflow in upper 17 generations of human respiratory tract. Journal of Biomechanics. 2008;**41**:2047-2054

[8] Tgavalekos NT, Venegas JG, Suki B, Lutchen KR. Relation between structure, function, and imaging in a three-dimensional model of the lung. Annals of Biomedical Engineering. 2003;**31**:363-373

[9] Musante CJ, Martonen TB. Computer simulations of particle deposition in the developing human lung. Journal of the Air & Waste Management Association. 2000;**50**:1426-1432

[10] Weibel ER, Taylor RC. Design and structure of the human lung. In: Fishman AP, editor. Pulmonary Diseases and Disorders. Vol. 1. New York: McGraw-Hill; 1988. pp. 11-60

[11] Landau LD, Lifshitz EM. Fluid Mechanics. London: Pergamon Press; 1987. 548 p

[12] ICRP. Human respiratory tract model for radiological protection. International Commission on RadiologicalProtection (ICRP) Publication 66. Annals of the ICRP. 1994;**24**:1-3

[13] NCRP. Deposition retention and dosimetry of inhaled radioactive substances. National Council on Radiation Protection and Measurements (NCRP). NCRP Report. 1997;**125**

[14] Kabilan S, Lin CL, Hoffman EA. Characteristics of airflow in a CT-based ovine lung: A numerical study. Journal of Applied Physiology. 2007;**102**: 1469-1482

[15] Caro C. Swirling steady inspiratory flow in models of human bronchial airways. Annals of Biomedical Engineering. 2001;**29**:138-149

[16] Comer JK, Kleinstreuer C, Zhang Z. Flow structures and particle deposition patterns in double-bifurcation airway models. Part 1. Air flow fields. Journal of Fluid Mechanics. 2001;**435**:25-54

[17] Ayinde TF. A generalized relationship for swirl decay in laminar pipe flow. Sadhana. 2010;**35**(Part 2): 129-137

Chapter 9

The Immunology of Asthma and Allergic Rhinitis

Andrew Kiboneka and Dan Kibuule

Abstract

The immune system is a complex collection of cells, tissues, and chemical mediators positioned throughout the body, whose primary purpose is to protect us against infection. However, its function is not only fundamental in protection from infectious disease but also provides aberrant response in allergens such as with asthma and allergic rhinitis. Allergic diseases like asthma and allergic rhinitis are characterized by a distinct type of inflammatory response, driven by immunoglobulin E (IgE)-dependent mechanisms. In asthma and allergic rhinitis, the inflammatory response is mediated by interaction of several immune cells (monocytes, lymphocytes, and polymorphonuclear cells) and cellular chemical mediators. In particular, atopic allergic response leads to destruction of multiple target cells such as epithelial, parenchymal and vascular and connective tissue of the airways. In addition, in inflammatory response in asthma and allergic rhinitis, sensory nerves are sensitized, leading to clinical manifestations. Sneezing and coughing are hypersensitivity responses of sensory nerves in allergic rhinitis and asthma, respectively. Similarly, nasal congestion and discharge in allergic rhinitis are due to vasodilatation that leads to plasma exudates as well as mucous secretion. The allergic inflammatory response is regulated by several transcription factors, particularly nuclear factor-κb (NF-κB), GATA-3 protein 3, and GATA binding protein.

Keywords: immunology, asthma and allergic rhinitis,, TH2 high, TH2 low, IL2 cells, Clara cell secretory protein (CC16), thymic stromal lymphopoietin (TSLP), interleukin (IL)-33, phenotypes, endotypes, united airway hypothesis, biological agents

1. Introduction

Allergic responses are mediated by IgE, a type of antibody associated with mast cells and basophils [1, 2]. Allergic rhinitis (i.e., inflammation of epithelia of nostril) is a reaction to allergens in the environment such as dust, pollen grain, and animal dander, among others. Patients with allergic rhinitis often present with congestion and inflammation (i.e., pain, reddening, and swelling) of the mucous membranes of the upper respiratory tract (nose, throat, eyes, and ears). In contrast, asthma is a complex heterogeneous syndrome characterized by increased inflammatory cells, airway hyper-reactivity (AHR), and structural changes in the lung [3]. The histological features of asthma include edema, cellular infiltration (typically with a prominent T lymphocyte and an eosinophil component), and sub-basement membrane collagen deposition.

Asthma is defined according to the Global Initiative for Asthma (GINA) 2018 as a heterogeneous disease, usually characterized by chronic airway inflammation.

Asthma is induced by an inflammatory response against usually manageable environmental inorganic and organic compounds in the respiratory tract. Indeed, asthma attacks can be triggered by exercise, viral illness, and allergens such as pollen. Other triggers include medications, extremes of weather, stress, smoke, and certain foods. Key indicators include a history of respiratory symptoms such as wheeze, shortness of breath, chest tightness, and cough that vary over time and in intensity, together with variable expiratory airflow limitation. It has variations in severity, natural history, and response to therapy [4].

Patients diagnosed with atopy have an increased likelihood to allergic responses mediated via IgE, mast cells, and CD4+ lymphocytes. In atopy, the allergic inflammatory responses are mainly due to cytokines (interleukins (IL-3, IL-4, and IL-5)) released from CD4+ lymphocytes. The interleukins increase the IgE production to neutralize the allergens. However, the binding of IgE-allergen complex formed further induces de novo synthesis and release of vasoactive substances that exacerbate the inflammatory reaction. This allergic inflammatory response occurs in two stages (early and late response) in both asthma and allergic rhinitis.

The allergic immune response recognizes allergens via germ line or random encoding, which can be innate and adaptive. The innate allergic immune responses are the first line of defense against allergens that use germ-line encoding and phagocytic cells. In contrast, the adaptive allergic response is mainly designed against infection and allergenic proteins from weed and pollen.

1.1 Pathogenesis of allergic rhinitis and asthma

According to the World Health Organization (WHO), the burden of asthma is estimated to have 300 million cases worldwide, making it one of the commonest noncommunicable diseases. Asthma is a serious global health problem affecting all age groups, with increasing prevalence in developing countries, treatment costs, and a burden for patients and the community. The WHO ranks asthma the highest among chronic illnesses afflicting the pediatric population worldwide. Of concern is that the majority of case fatalities attributed to asthma occur among populations in underdeveloped countries characterized with weak health systems for control and management of the disease [4–7].

Whereas allergic rhinitis results from activation of mucosal mast cells, asthma is triggered by allergen activation of submucosal mast cells in the lower airways. The nature and development airway inflammation may be driven by numerous factors, including pathogenic infections, pollution, or even relatively innocuous inhaled particles, such as allergens. International guidelines are available for the management of severe asthma by the European Respiratory Society and the American Thoracic Society [6].

Chronic allergen exposure leads to the continuous presence of increased number of lymphocytes, eosinophils, neutrophils, basophils, and other leukocytes causing airway hyper-reactivity and remodeling—a thickening of the airway walls due to hyperplasia and hypertrophy of the smooth muscle layer, with the eventual development of fibrosis.

It has become apparent that there are many phenotypic and endotype types of asthma. In patients with allergic asthma endotypes, allergen can cause activation of mast cells in an antigen-specific manner. Also allergens can stimulate the airway epithelium, through toll-like receptors (TLRs) and other damage receptors, to release IL-25, IL33, and thymic stromal lymphopoietin (TSLP). These cytokines can lead to the activation of submucosal type two innate lymphoid cells (ILC2), inducing these to release IL-4, IL-5, IL-9, and IL-13.

2. Methodology

A comprehensive review of all aspects of immunology, components of the immune system, immune responses to asthma and allergic rhinitis in children and adults, and airway epithelial cell mucosal immunology was done in a systematic and explicit search of PubMed and HINARI—identifying, selecting, and critically appraising relevant research and textbooks of Immunology from Europe and the United States of America used in undergraduate and postgraduate Medical Education (Cochrane Collaboration) [7–9].

3. Results/findings

Critical analysis of scientific concepts in pulmonary immune inflammation of asthma and allergic rhinitis and an analysis of similarities, differences, and interactions between these two diseases are done.

Knowledge of our immune system functions is critical in understanding allergic airway disease development as well as for selection of appropriate diagnostic and therapeutic options for patients with asthma and allergic rhinitis. A robust inflammatory response is essential to control asthma and allergic rhinitis, and both active and innate mechanisms of immunity are important in this regard. The failure of resolution or persistent pro-inflammatory immune responses results in chronic inflammatory airway diseases like asthma and allergic rhinitis. It is also becoming increasingly important to phenotype airway inflammation in individual patients to allow targeted treatment as we move toward personalized therapies for asthma.

The majority of patients of asthma suffer from an allergic variant of the disease that is triggered by an IgE-driven immune response directed against inhaled antigens and leads to various symptoms, such as wheezing, coughing, and breathing difficulties. The immunopathogenesis of allergic asthma involves a complex interplay between the immune system and parenchymal cells of the lung, including the airway epithelium [10, 11].

Inhaled allergens are phagocytosed by macrophages and dendritic cells (DCs) presented on major histocompatibility complex (MHC) class II molecules and initiate the differentiation of Th2 cells and a humoral immune response. Following class switching, Ag-specific B cells secrete immunoglobulin E which causes degranulation of mast cells.

Cytokines, such as IL-4, IL-5, and IL-13, are produced by TH2 cells, mast cells, basophils, and type 2 innate lymphoid cells, as well as airway epithelial cells, and they trigger pathological events, including airway wall remodeling, bronchial hyper responsiveness, and goblet cell metaplasia. Once the immune response has been initiated, eosinophils become the major effector cells that are responsible for airway dysfunction. In addition to the importance of immune cells in allergic asthma, there is evidence for a prominent role of airway epithelial cells in this disease (**Table 1**).

3.1 The innate inflammatory immune response and asthma/cells of the immune system

Innate immunity is the body's immediate response to an infection. It is a non-specific response, meaning that the same response is mounted to a large number of different pathogens. When activated, the innate response is often seen as an inflammatory response. Inflammation is the body's response to injury or tissue damage.

	Pulmonary immune cell types/ receptors	Summary of functions
A. Innate immune system	Phagocytic cells (polymorphonuclear cells, monocyte-macrophages, and eosinophils) Dendritic cells Mast cells Eosinophils Basophils Pattern recognition receptors TREG cell Natural killer cells NKT cells IL2 cells	Airway dendritic cells (DC) are critical mediators of immune responses in the lung by virtue of their ability to sample, process, and present inhaled antigens to T cells
B. Adaptive immune response	T and B cells	
C. Bronchial epithelial cells	• Clara cells • Ciliated cells • Goblet cells	The interleukins IL-25 and IL-33 and thymic stromal lymphopoietin are produced by injured epithelium and play critical roles in driving expression of Th2 cytokines

Table 1.
Classification of the immune system, immune cells, and the inflammatory response in asthma summary of functions.

Phagocytic cells are a part of the innate immune system and consist of polymorphonuclear cells, monocytes-macrophages, and eosinophils. Neutrophils and monocytes are normally found circulating in the bloodstream and are recruited to sites of infection by the process of extravasation. Receptors on the phagocyte interact with ligands on vascular endothelium, and the cells attach, arrest, and move from the circulation to the diseased tissue/lungs.

Monocytes, similar to neutrophils, can also migrate into the tissues and on doing so differentiate into macrophages. Macrophages have a number of key functions, including phagocytosis of infecting microbes, antigen presentation, and general removal of dying or damaged host cells [12].

3.1.1 Dendritic cells

These are bone marrow-derived cells, found in most tissues, including lymphoid tissues. Discovered by Ralph Steinman in the mid-1970s, dendritic cells are critical for the initiation of the immune response. They are so named, because of being covered with long membranous extensions that resemble the dendrites (extensions) of the nerve cells.

Dendritic cells capture antigens, e.g., pollen/animal dander, and process these antigens and then present them to naive T cells, initiating the adaptive immune response. The first stage of an immune response to any antigen is the processing and presentation of that antigen by antigen-presenting cells (APCs), e.g., dendritic cells.

3.1.2 Pattern recognition receptors (PRRs)

These are receptors of the innate immune system that recognize common molecular patterns on pathogen surfaces called pathogen-associated molecular patterns (PAMPS), structures that are conserved in broad classes of pathogens for their functional importance. Many of these receptors reside at the plasma membrane. They are proteins expressed, mainly, by cells of the innate immune system, such as dendritic cells, macrophages, monocytes, neutrophils, and epithelial cells.

i. One group of receptors, **C-type lectins**, recognizes certain sugar units that are typically located at the terminal position of carbohydrate chains on pathogen surfaces.

ii. Another group and one of the best-characterized signaling PRR families is the evolutionary conserved **toll-like receptor system** in mammals, named after a homologous receptor system used by the *Drosophila* fruit fly for protection from infection. In humans, there are 10 expressed TLR genes in mice [13], their products forming homo- or heterodimers with other family members, thus increasing the repertoire for recognition. TLR4, for example, has been shown to be the receptor recognizing lipopolysaccharide (LPS) found on the surface of Gram-negative bacteria such as *Escherichia coli* but not present on mammalian cells. The effect of pathogen components binding to TLRs on innate immune cells is TLR activation, which initiates signaling into the immune cell and the increased expression of a large number of target genes. The genes involved depend on the pattern of TLRs engaged, but common outcomes include the increased production of inflammatory mediators such as cytokines and chemokines, enhanced phagocytosis (internalization and killing of the pathogen), upregulation of costimulatory molecules on the cell surface, cell migration, and, in the case of macrophages, increased processing and presentation of pathogen antigens to activate an adaptive immune response.

There are also three other families of receptors that sense PAMPS when pathogens arrive in the cytoplasm:

i. NOD-like receptors (NLRs): e.g., NOD1 and NOD2

ii. RIG-like helicases (RLHs): the cytoplasmic RNA-helicase, RIG-I, and related proteins act as virus receptors

iii. Cyclic GMP-AMP synthase (cGAS, cGAMP synthase): NB

Functions of NOD1 and NOD2 and cyclic GMP-AMP synthase:

- NLRs is an acronym that stands for NOD-like receptors. These are a large family of cytosolic proteins activated by intracellular PAMPS. NOD1 and NOD2 recognize important PAMPS, e.g., muramyl dipeptides produced during the synthesis or degradation of either intracellular or extracellular bacteria.

- cGMP-AMP (cGAMP) synthase (cGAS) is a cytosolic DNA sensor that activates innate immune responses.

3.1.3 Mast cells

A large granule-rich cell found in the connective tissue of the body, most abundantly in the submucosal tissues and the dermis. The granules store bioactive molecules including the vasoactive amine, which are released on mast cell-activated and are involved in the pathogenesis of bronchoconstriction in asthmatic airways [13, 14].

3.1.4 Eosinophils

A type of white blood cell containing granules that stain with eosin and is an effector cell in asthma as well as produces cytokines, e.g., IL-5 [15, 16]. In the airway of asthmatic patients, eosinophil-derived mediators of inflammation, including eosinophil-derived neurotoxin (EDN), major basic protein (MBP), and lysophospholipase (LPL), are toxic to the respiratory epithelium contributing to the immune pathogenesis of asthma in both children and adults [16].

3.1.5 Basophils

A type of white blood cell containing granules that stain with basic dyes. Basophils are non-phagocytic granulocytes. In response to binding of circulating antibodies, basophils release their contents including histamine which cause smooth muscle contraction in asthmatic airways as well as increasing blood permeability which may account for edema of the airways in asthma and inflammation [17, 18]. Basophils and mast cells release mediators of immediate hypersensitivity, e.g., histamine. Basophils are present in the blood stream, whereas mast cells are present only in the tissue.

3.1.6 Natural killer cells

A type of innate lymphoid cell (ILC) that is important in innate immunity to viruses and other intracellular pathogens and in antibody-dependent cellular cytotoxicity (ADCC) hypersensitivity reacyions.

They do not express antigen receptors and are considered part of the innate immune system, despite being lymphoid cells [19, 20].

3.1.7 NKT cells

Is another type of cell in the lymphoid lineage that shares features with both conventional T lymphocytes and NK cells like T cells; NKT cells have T-cell receptors (TCRs) and some express CD4. Unlike most T cells, however, the TCRs of NKT cells are not very diverse and recognize specific lipids and glycolipids presented by a molecule related to the major histocompatibility complex (MHC) proteins called CD1.

Like their innate immune counterparts, NK cells, NKT cells have antibody receptors.

NKT cells are considered as a cell subset belonging to the innate immune system with the capacity to amplify adaptive immune responses in asthma [7–9, 21].

Defining the roles of thymic stromal lymphopoietin, IL-25, and IL-3 in human asthma:

IL-25, IL-33, and TLSP are epithelial-derived cytokines and have been identified as having an important role in asthma pathogenesis. These cytokines have been described as epithelial-derived alarmins that activate and potentiate the innate and humoral arms of the immune system in the presence of actual or perceived damage.

TSLP is increased in asthmatic airways, mast cells and in the lungs is produced mainly by airway epithelial cells. In addition, these three cytokines can generate a H2 cytokine profile independent of the adaptive immune system. TSLP is a

TH2-promoting cytokine that significantly contributes to the immune pathogenesis of asthma [22–24].

3.1.8 IL-33

Interleukin-33 (IL-33), which belongs to the larger family of damage-associated molecular pattern molecules, has been considered as an "alarmin" [22–24]. It is released to alert the immune system by first-line cells, such as tissue epithelial cells.

3.1.9 IL-C2

Innate lymphoid cells are a group of lymphoid cells with a recently recognized role as regulators of innate immunity, inflammation, and tissue repair at the barrier surfaces. They are a lymphoid subclass characterized by the lack of either B- or T-cell receptors but retain cytotoxic or immunomodulatory capacity [22–24].

The innate defense system contains cells that look just like B or T lymphocytes under the microscope, yet express neither B- nor T-cell receptors. These cells are known as innate lymphoid cells.

Innate lymphoid cells are classified into three groups based on their transcription factors and cytokine production patterns, which mirror helper T-cell subsets. Unlike T cells and B cells, ILCs do not have antigen receptors. They respond to innate factors released by the bronchial epithelium, such as cytokines and alarmins, including IL-33, IL-25, and thymic stromal lymphopoietin [22–24]. ILCs produce multiple pro-inflammatory and immune regulatory cytokines for the induction and regulation of inflammation.

3.1.10 CC16 club cells/Clara cells

Clara cells are non-ciliated, non-mucous, secretory cells in respiratory epithelium. These epithelial cells secrete several distinctive proteins, including Clara cell 10-kDa secretory protein (CCSP). Clara cells are most predominant in the terminal and respiratory bronchioles of humans.

Club cells, also known as bronchiolar exocrine cells and originally known as Clara cells, are dome-shaped cells with short microvilli, found in the small airways (bronchioles) of the lungs.

Of recent Clara cells (CC16) have re-emerged in the immune pathogenesis of Asthma [25].

3.2 The adaptive inflammatory cells

T-cell responses to antigens consist of a combination of pro-inflammatory (effector) and anti-inflammatory (regulatory) cells.

- Lymphocytes differentiate into separate lineages. The B lymphocytes secrete antibodies.

The T lymphocytes operate in a supervising role to mediate cellular and humoral responses. Antigen presentation describes a vital immune process which is essential for T-cell immune response triggering immunity. B and T lymphocytes produce and express specific receptors for antigens. Collectively, the functions of the T and B cells encompass an entity called the adaptive immune system.

T-helper lymphocytes conventionally are TH1 and TH2 cells. TH1 cells produce cytokines that downregulate the atopic response. In those who are genetically susceptible to developing asthma, antigen presentation to T-helper cells leads to a

TH2 response, pro-inflammatory cytokines, and upregulation of airway inflammation of asthma by enhancing immunoglobulin E synthesis, eosinophils, and mast cell activation/function.

3.2.1 TREG cells

TREG cells, a type of T-helper lymphocytes, bind interleukins 2 via the CD25 and CD45RB receptors to signal suppression of the immune system. This is essential in arresting inflammatory allergic responses such as in asthma and allergic rhinitis. In addition, naive T lymphocytes are induced to synthesize FoxP3 which acts as a transcription factor for the cytokines involved in the TREG-mediated cascade. In particular, transforming growth factor-β (TGF-β) and interleukin-10 are the main cytokines implicated in the TREG-mediated suppression of inflammatory allergic responses [26, 27]. Thus, TREG cells are critical in the autoregulation of allergic inflammatory reactions by slowing the pathological effects of the Th2 type immune responses in bronchial hyper-reactivity and inflammation in asthma [26–28].

3.3 The respiratory airway cells/mucosal immunology

There are several cells in the epithelium of the lower respiratory tract. The upper part includes support cells (basement), mucous-secreting cells, and the cilia, to aid the expulsion of mucous. However, Clara cells and cilia dominate in the lower parts of the respiratory system [29, 30].

Some of these cells are involved in inflammatory allergic responses in asthma. For instance, in asthma the goblet cells, i.e., mucous-secreting cells, increased the number of goblet cells as part of airway remodeling. The mucus (i.e., a complex solution of lipids and proteins in the airways) aggravates the immunopathology of asthma. The function of mucous is to trap inhaled particles/allergen and the interaction with the tips of beating cilia and remove particles/allergen from the airways, a process termed mucociliary clearance [31]. Other cells such as the neuroendocrine cells are not directly involved in the immunopathogenesis of asthma. Neuroendocrine cells (i.e., small round cells with dark staining nucleus and clear cytoplasm) contain characteristic granules and secrete hormones and peptides such as serotonin.

In particular, lymphoid tissues are mainly found in the bronchial. Thus during an asthmatic attack, the airways are remodeled (i.e., bronchial thermoplasty), which is characterized by swelling, cellular infiltration, and hyperplasia of smooth muscles and goblet cells [7–9].

The adaptation (i.e., hypertrophy, metaplasia, fibrosis, and hyperplasia) of the epithelial airways and smooth muscle cells to allergic and/or noxious stimuli compromises the structure and function of the airways [31, 32].

Indeed, the epithelial cells are important in providing rapid response to counter allergens by secreting mucous and initiating the inflammation. This epithelium provides a barrier against the external environment and protects against infection from airborne pathogens. Defective barrier function or viral infection can lead to respiratory tract disease like asthma.

The first line of defense against invasion by potential pathogens is the thin layer of epithelium that covers mucosal surfaces including that of the upper and lower respiratory tract. The mucosal immune system has unique features including large size, uptake, and presentation of antigen and contains a large number of effector T lymphocytes. The circulation of lymphocytes within the mucosal immune system is controlled by tissue-specific adhesion molecules and chemokine receptors.

The analysis of molecular markers of airway inflammation has provided promising and noninvasive techniques that facilitate the detection of disease phenotypes as well as measurement of therapeutic efficacy for asthma.

Current treatments for severe forms of asthma have been extended to the use of biological modifiers for the classical asthma endotypes (i.e., Th2 high and Th2 low). Conventional immune modulators (omalizumab, mepolizumab, reslizumab, benralizumab, and dupilumab) used in the management of severe forms of asthma are for patients with asthma of the type Th2 high. The inflammatory in patients with TH2 high asthma is principally mediated by eosinophils reactions as well as type 2 cytokines (i.e., IL-4, IL-13, IL-5) produced by Th2 cells. The type 2 cytokines are in turn regulated by other interleukins, namely, IL-25 and IL-33, as well as TSLP [9, 10]. These mediators are upstream innate factors that drive IL-13 and IL-5 production.

In contrast, TH2 low asthma is poorly described. Patients do not have eosinophilia and other markers but have neutrophilia inflammation. This is mainly due to the activation of TH1 or 17 cells that release IFN and IL-17. These cells are specifically produced at mucosal surfaces and thus are important in airway inflammation. The role of ILCs, more specifically type 2 ILCs, in the pathogenesis of allergic airway diseases has been extensively investigated over the last decade. Chronic nasal inflammation may aggravate or lead to the development of other significant disorders, including asthma, rhinosinusitis, and middle ear disease.

3.3.1 Allergic rhinitis and mediators of the inflammatory response

Sensitization is initiated in nasal tissues when antigen that is deposited on the nasal mucosa is engulfed by antigen-presenting cells—macrophages, dendritic cells, Langerhans cells—and partially degraded within their phagolysosomes into antigenic peptides. These peptides are then externalized on the surfaces of APCs and are presented to naive CD4+ T lymphocytes. The interaction of T-helper lymphocytes is activated by presentation of an allergen via the MHC class II receptor on macrophages and other cells [32–34].

In patients with allergic rhinitis, allergen-triggered early and late responses are mediated by a series of inflammatory cells. Within minutes of contact with allergen, IgE-sensitized mast cells degranulate, releasing both preformed and newly synthesized mediators. Immunologic processes in both nasal and bronchial tissues involve TH2 lymphocytes and eosinophils. Eosinophils are the predominant cell in the chronic inflammatory process characteristic of the late-phase allergic response. Eosinophils release an array of pro-inflammatory mediators, including cysteinyl leukotrienes, cationic proteins, eosinophil peroxidase, and major basic protein, and might serve as a major source of IL-3, IL-5, GM-CSF, and IL-13. Neuropeptides also appear to contribute to the pathophysiology of allergic rhinitis symptoms.

3.3.2 Allergen exposure

The respiratory tract is an important route of allergen entry. Several people react to airborne allergens with an IgE-mediated reaction, resulting from the deposition of mucosal mast cells beneath the nasal epithelium by allergens such as pollen that when they contact the epithelium, they release their soluble protein content, which is rich in eosinophils and allergic rhinitis characterized by intense itching, sneezing, nasal blockage, and irritation of the nasal mucosa due to histamine release.

In atopic-related allergic rhinitis, the hypersensitivity mediated via IgE, mast cells, and lymphocytes is inherited. The continued exposure of allergens initiates the inflammatory process via the APC, lymphocytes, and cytokine cascades (i.e., IL-3, IL-4, and IL-5). Until, then the immune system is not yet sensitized to the allergen. Following sensitization, further exposures initiate the inflammatory/allergic response and clinical presentation of allergic rhinitis.

3.3.3 United airway hypothesis/disease

Upper and lower airways are considered a unified morphological and functional unit, and the connection existing between them has been observed for many years, both in health and in disease [35]. The respiratory system is integrated, and thus the allergic diseases of the lower (i.e., asthma) and the upper respiratory tract (allergic rhinitis) have similar pathogenesis and should be considered as one. Indeed, precious studies have shown an overlap in the clinical presentation of these two diseases where patients with allergic rhinitis are at risk for asthma.

4. Conclusions

Asthma and allergic rhinitis are a complex heterogeneous group of airway diseases that affects both children and adults worldwide. Through the use of molecular and cellular immunology, conceptual shifts have been made in the understanding of these diseases involving both innate and adaptive immunity as well examination of airway epithelial changes that occur with asthma, evolving into personalized-targeted therapy for asthma in view of these mechanisms. Allergic rhinitis is the most common of all atopic diseases, and although it can develop at any age, most patients report the onset of symptoms before 30 years of age, making it the most common chronic disorder in children.

Acknowledgements

i. Professor Russel Hopp. Omaha. Nebraska, USA (tutor during allergy/immunology fellowship at Creighton University, Omaha, Nebraska, USA)

ii. Professor Peter Nyarango. Dean. School of Medicine. University of Namibia. Windhoek, Namibia

Conflict of interest

No conflict of interest to declare.

Thanks

i. To my wife Priscilla and children Valeria, Rhonah, Ronnie, and Victoria (for their loving support and encouragement).

ii. To my parents Dr. and Mrs. Gad Kiboneka (for their inspiration and educating me).

Author details

Andrew Kiboneka[1*] and Dan Kibuule[2]

1 Department of Pediatrics, School of Medicine, Faculty of Health Sciences, University of Namibia, Windhoek, Namibia

2 Department of Pharmacy Practice and Policy, School of Pharmacy, Faculty of Health Sciences, University of Namibia, Windhoek, Namibia

*Address all correspondence to: akiboneka@yahoo.com; akiboneka@unam.na

References

[1] Wallace DV, Dykewicz MS, Bernstein DI, Blessing-Moore J, Cox L, Khan DA, et al. The diagnosis and management of rhinitis: An updated practice parameter. The Journal of Allergy and Clinical Immunology. 2008;**122**:S1-S84. 18662584

[2] Blaiss MS, Dykewicz MS, Skoner DP, Smith N, Leatherman B, Craig TJ, et al. Diagnosis and treatment of nasal and ocular allergies: The Allergies, Immunotherapy, and RhinoconjunctivitiS (AIRS) surveys. Annals of Allergy, Asthma & Immunology. 2014;**112**:322-328

[3] Lötvall J et al. Asthma endotypes: A new approach to classification of disease entities within the asthma syndrome. The Journal of Allergy and Clinical Immunology. 2011;**127**(2):355-360

[4] Global Initiative for Asthma. Available from: http://www.ginasthma.org/guidelines-gina-report-global-strategy-for-asthma

[5] National Asthma Education and Prevention Program Expert Panel Report 3. Guidelines for the Diagnosis and Management of Asthma; Summary Report 2007

[6] Reddel HK, Taylor DR, Bateman ED, et al. An official American Thoracic Society/European Respiratory Society statement. Asthma control and exacerbations: Standardizing endpoints for clinical asthma trials and clinical practice. American Journal of Respiratory and Critical Care Medicine. 2009;**180**:59-99

[7] Abbas AK et al. Cellular and Molecular Immunology. 7th ed. Philadelphia, USA, Saunders: Elsevier; 2012

[8] Owen JA, Punt J, Stranford SA Jones P, Kuby J. Immunology. 7th ed. New York: W.H Freeman, Macmillan Learning; 2013

[9] Leung DYM et al. Pediatric Allergy. Principles and Practice. 3rd ed. E-Book. USA: Elsevier Health Sciences; 2010

[10] Crystal RG et al. Airway epithelial cells. Current concepts and challenges. Proceedings of the American Thoracic Society. 2008;**5**:772-777

[11] Erle DJ, Sheppard D. The cell biology of asthma. The Journal of Cell Biology. 2014;**205**(5):621-631

[12] Holgate ST. Innate and adaptive immune responses in asthma. Nature Medicine. 2012;**18**:673-683

[13] Galli SJ, Nakae, et al. Mast cells in the development of adaptive immune responses. Nature Immunology. 2005;**6**:135-142

[14] Taube C et al. The leukocyte B4 receptor (BLT1) is required for effective CD+T cell mediated airway hype responsiveness. Journal of Immunology. 2006;**176**:3157-3164

[15] Blanchard C et al. Biology of the eosinophil. Advances in Immunology. 2009;**101**:81-82

[16] Hogan SP et al. Eosinophils: Biological properties and role in health and disease. Clinical & Experimental Allergy. May 2008;**38**(5):709-750

[17] MacGlashan D et al. Basophils in airway disease. Current Allergy and Asthma Reports. 2002;**2**:126-132

[18] Schwartz C. Basophils in inflammation. European Journal of Pharmacology. 2016;**778**:90-95

[19] Vivier E et al. Functions of natural killer cells. Nature Immunology. 2008;**9**:503-510

[20] Vivier E et al. Innate or adaptive immunity? The example of natural killer cells. Science. 2011;**331**:44-49

[21] Abbas AK et al. Basic Immunology. Functions and Disorders of the Immune Syste. 4th ed. Philadelphia, USA, Saunders: Elsevier; 2014

[22] Defining the roles of IL-33, thymic stromal lymphopoietin, and IL-25 in human asthma. American Journal of Respiratory and Critical Care Medicine. 2014;**190**(7):715-721

[23] Vannella KM et al. Combinatorial targeting of TSLP, IL-25, and IL-33 in type 2 cytokine-driven inflammation and fibrosis. Science Translational Medicine. 2016;**8**(337):337ra65

[24] Divekar R et al. Recent advances in epithelium-derived cytokines (IL-33, IL-25 and TSLP) and allergic inflammation. Current Opinion in Allergy and Clinical Immunology. 2015;**15**(1):98-103

[25] Sonar SS et al. Clara cells drive eosinophil accumulation in allergic asthma. The European Respiratory Journal. 2012;**39**(2):429-438

[26] Sakguchi S et al. Regulatory T cells and immune tolerance. Cell. 2008;**133**:775-787

[27] Sagakuchi S. Naturally occurring Foxp3 expressing CD25+, CD4+ regulatory T cells in immunologic tolerance to self & non-self. Nature Immunology. 2005;**6**:345-352

[28] Saraiva M et al. The regulation of IL-10 production by immune cells. Nature Reviews Immunology. 2010;**10**(3):170-181

[29] Lambrecht BN et al. Allergens and the airway epithelium response: Gateway to allergic sensitization. The Journal of Allergy and Clinical Immunology. 1 Sep 2014;**134**(3):499-507

[30] Adkinson Jr NF, Bochner BS, Burks AW, Busse WW, Holgate ST, Lemanske RF, O'Hehir, RE. Middleton's allergy E-Book: Principles and practice. USA: Elsevier Health Sciences; 18 Sep 2013

[31] Fahy JV. Remodeling of the airway epithelium in asthma. American Journal of Respiratory and Critical Care Medicine. 2001;**164**:S46-S51

[32] Bugeon L, Dallman M. Costimulation of T cells. American Journal of Respiratory and Critical Care Medicine. 2000;**162**:S164-S168 11029388

[33] Liu YJ. IPC: Professional type 1 interferon-producing cells and plasmacytoid dendritic cell precursors. Annual Review of Immunology. 2005;**23**:275-306 15771572

[34] Bharadwaj AS, Bewtra AK, Agrawal DK. Dendritic cells in allergic airway inflammation. Canadian Journal of Physiology and Pharmacology. 2007;**85**:686-699

[35] Giavina-Bianchi P et al. United airway disease: Current perspectives. Journal of Asthma and Allergy. 2016;**9**:93-100

Section 5

Surgical Techniques in Sino-Nasal Diseases

Chapter 10

Turbinate Surgery in Chronic Rhinosinusitis: Techniques and Ultrastructural Outcomes

Giampiero Neri, Fiorella Cazzato, Elisa Vestrini, Pasquina La Torre, Giampaolo Quaternato, Letizia Neri and Lucia Centurione

Abstract

Chronic nasal obstruction due to hypertrophic rhinitis is commonly associated with perennial allergic and nonallergic rhinitis. It is not a simple enlargement of mucosal and submucosal tissues, but it is characterized by deep histological modifications. This pathology, a very frequent condition encountered in rhinological practice, has a significant impact on quality of life. Patients usually complain about sneezing, rhinorrhea, frontal headache, postnasal drip, snoring, blocked nasal ducts, and sleep disorders. When medical therapy fails, surgical reduction of inferior turbinates is mandatory. A large variety of surgical techniques in literature exist, but there is a lack of consensus about which is the proper technique to perform. In this chapter, we describe the most important techniques of inferior turbinate reduction with advantages and disadvantages of each one.

Keywords: turbinate hypertrophy, nasal obstruction, nasal surgery, techniques, turbinoplasty

1. Introduction

Chronic nasal obstruction is a very frequent condition in rhinological practice that severely interferes with the quality of life [1]. The most common cause of this complaint is chronic hypertrophic rhinitis. It consists of a chronical swelling of the inferior turbinate [2].

Turbinate hypertrophy, commonly associated with perennial allergic and nonallergic rhinitis [1], is not a simple enlargement of mucosal and submucosal tissues, but it is characterized by deep histological modifications such as severe damage of the epithelial barrier, disappearance of ciliated and goblet cells, inflammatory infiltration of the lamina propria, fibrosis, prominent venous congestion, and basement membrane interruption [2].

Patients generally complain about sneezing, rhinorrhea, postnasal drip, frontal headache, blocked nasal passages, sleep disturbance, and snoring [3].

When medical treatment with topical corticosteroids, antihistamines, and decongestants fails, surgical reduction of inferior turbinates could be attempted.

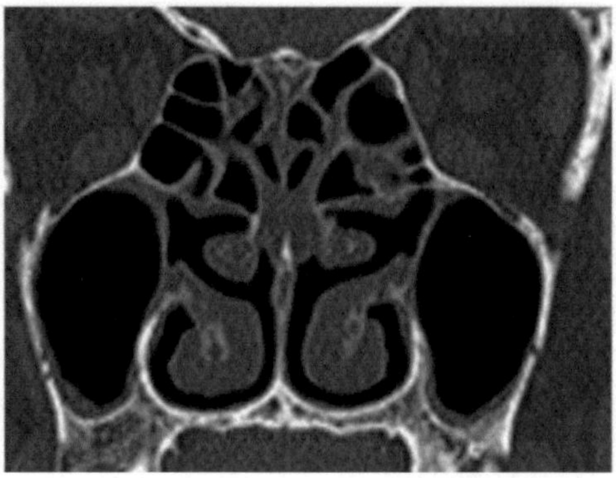

Figure 1.
The radiologic study with head-CT shows a normal anatomy of the turbinates and the nasosinusal system.

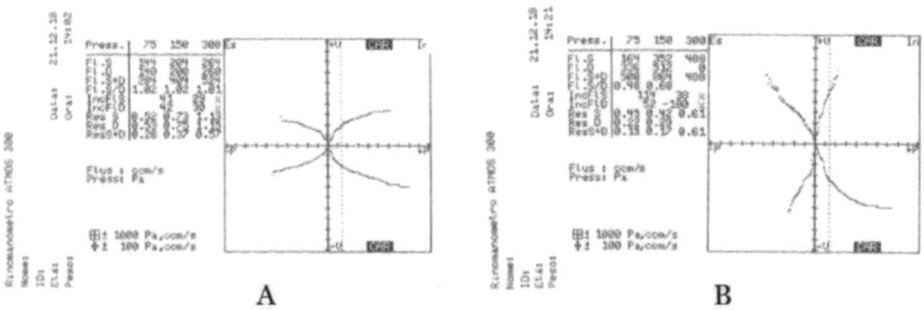

Figure 2.
Rhinomanometric evaluation before (A) and after (B) application of nasal topical decongestant shows the improvement of respiratory nasal flux.

The goal of turbinate surgery is to improve nasal patency by minimizing complications such us postoperative hemorrhage, crusting, foul odor, and the "empty nose syndrome" [4].

There is a variety of turbinate procedures, but there is a lack of consensus about which technique is the best [5].

Turbinate hypertrophy can be divided into primary and secondary. The primary hypertrophy is related to the submucosal component, while the secondary hypertrophy is due to contralateral septal deviation and is related to the bony component of the turbinate. It is important to distinguish these two types of hypertrophy in order to decide the proper procedure to perform. The anatomic radiologic study (**Figure 1**) and the rhinomanometric evaluation (**Figure 2**) are mandatory for surgical indication [6].

2. Surgical techniques

Turbinate reduction techniques can be divided into four categories [7]:

1. Extramucosal debulking procedures

2. Superficial extramucosal procedures

3. Dislocation procedures

4. Submucosal procedures

2.1 Extramucosal debulking procedures

These procedures include:

1. Total turbinectomy

2. Partial turbinectomy

3. Microdebrider-assisted turbinoplasty (extramucosal technique)

2.1.1 Total turbinectomy

It is a technique that was described for the first time in the last 10 years of the nineteenth century. Jones in 1895 and Holmes in 1900 introduced the concept of total turbinectomy [8].

This technique is considered the most radical surgical technique on the inferior turbinate. After having fractured, the bone plate of the inferior turbinate (**Figure 3**), levering from the inferior meatus, with an angled scissors, the inferior turbinate is dissected for its entire length remaining adherent to the lateral wall of the nasal cavity.

For the immediate benefit that the patient obtains, it is often considered as safe and effective though its major complication is the possible bleeding, avoidable, however, both using adequate nasal swabs and avoiding to treat patients who take anticoagulants [9].

Unfortunately, this type of surgery, extremely aggressive, can later lead to dry nose syndrome or even the syndrome of the empty nose with a paradoxical obstruction. The obstructive event is due to the loss of normal nasal resistance and the formation of a laminar air column. This situation causes a poor contact between the air and the nasal walls, the mucosa, due to the absence of the sensory fibers of the inferior turbinate, shows a reduction or even a loss of the respiratory flow [6].

The altered aerodynamics pattern, due to total turbinectomy, generates many complications such as copious postoperative bleeding, quantitative reduction of the ciliary movement, mucosal dryness, and deficit of mucus clearance. All this

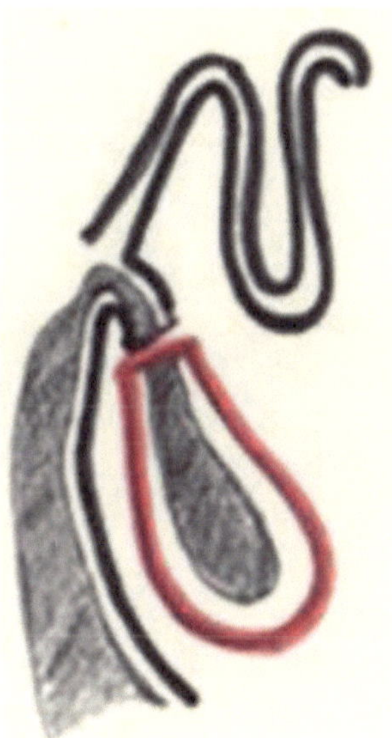

Figure 3.
Total turbinectomy.

creates stagnation of secretions, crusts formations (sometimes foul-smelling), and frequent infections with gradual development of dry inflammatory forms affecting the pharynx and larynx. Precisely because of its complications, this technique has now fallen into disuse [9].

TASCA states that it is wrong to transform the nasal cavities into rigid and inanimate tubes, unable to perform the functions of congestion and decongestion, depriving them of their natural function [10]; and for Huizing and de Groot, total turbinectomy is a nasal crime, and they do not consider it useful to perform the resection of more than a third or half of the inferior turbinate unless it is a tumor [11].

2.1.2 Partial turbinectomy

The partial turbinectomy (**Figure 4**) is used to limit the large surgical resections that are performed with total turbinectomy, and consists in the removal of the mucosa and bones of the anterior third of the inferior turbinate. The degree of resection is directly proportional to the degree of hypertrophy. Initially, the mucosal and the submucosal tissue are removed, and if there is bone hypertrophy, a small bone resection is also performed. There are several partial turbinectomy techniques.

The oldest technique is the crushing and trimming introduced by Kressner in 1930. Other technique is selective mucosotomy, which consists of the removal of the anterior or/and the posterior region of the turbinate following defined section lines. The diagonal resection consists in a sagittal exeresis with the purpose of preserving the head of the turbinate and eluting the posterior region of the turbinate. The horizontal resection of the inferior edge of the turbinate avoids the risk of bleeding from the sphenopalatine artery [12], which instead occurs in the diagonal resection [7].

The degloving technique was proposed by Chevretton et al. It consists of the resection of a large part of the turbinate, leaving the bone and the periosteum intact [7, 13].

TASCA et al. reported that the only appropriate techniques are "Crushing with remodeling" and "Resection of the tail." It is preferable to perform a resection of the posterior region of the inferior turbinate, because the elimination of the head of turbinate causes a great functional damage. It creates a deficit of the mucociliary clearance and the inferior turbinate loses its function of directing the inspiring currents [10].

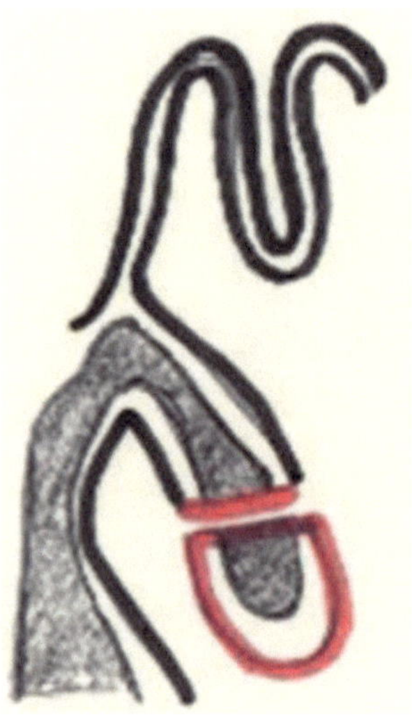

Figure 4.
Partial turbinectomy.

Crushing with remodeling is indicated if the hypertrophy is both anterior and posterior and allows to respect the functional capacity of the remaining portion of the turbinate. The turbinate is compressed using specific pliers and then reduced by cutting parallel or slightly diagonal strips starting from the lower edge. After the medial fracture of the turbinate performed with a smooth and chamfered instrument (the handle of a Cottle chisel can be used), it is squeezed with modified-Kressner tongs both anteriorly and posteriorly. The size of the turbinate is reduced by removing a strip from its rather flaccid bottom edge with Heymann-type scissors. If necessary, a part of bone is removed. Finally, the turbinate remaining laterally is repositioned. It is advised to perform a second surgical time if the hypertrophic tissue is excessive, avoiding to remove it in a single time [14].

Resection of degenerated tissue: if a part of the turbinate is damaged irreversibly, it is removed using long angled scissors or a loop [14].

Even if partial inferior turbinectomy is a simple and effective surgical procedure, it is equally troublesome if not performed correctly. Excessive resection of the inferior turbinate can lead to peri- or postoperative bleeding, from medial and inferior surface of the inferior turbinate, synechiae with the nasal septum and floor of nasal cavity, frequent post nasal blood drip, nasal crusting, and atrophic rhinitis. By using appropriate tools and limiting demolition, these complications can be avoided [15].

A study by Passali et al. demonstrated how the partial turbinectomy technique performed at the level of the inferior turbinate resolves most of the nasal obstruction. This technique however, even if minimally, causes damage to the nasal mucosa and therefore it is necessary that the surgeon is experienced to avoid complications [1, 16].

Sapci et al. reported that the use of radiofrequency to reduce hypertrophy of turbinates leads to an improvement of nasal obstruction and does not alter the ciliary mucus clearance. With the partial turbinectomy technique, the results obtained were similar to those of results with the radiofrequency tissue ablation technique [1, 17].

Salzano et al. enrolled four groups of patients each treated with radiofrequency, high-frequency electrocautery treatments, and lower partial turbinotomy to reduce the hypertrophied lower turbinates. They show that the partial inferior nasal turbinectomy is the best method of treatment, because it does not cause damage to the nasal mucosa or underlying sensibility nerves [18].

In the 1996, the microdebrider was first used by Davis and Nishioka to remove both medial and inferior redundant mucosal tissue and hypertrophied cavernous sinusoid of the inferior turbinate and the anterior head region of the inferior turbinate, up the superficial layer to the periosteum [19].

Generally, if the microdebrider-assisted turbinoplasty is limited to the decongestion of the turbinates only, the patient undergoes local anesthesia with vasoconstrictive drugs to create a large ischemia avoiding intraoperative bleeding. General anesthesia is necessary in the event that a septal or paranasal sinus surgery is also associated. In our experience, the local anesthesia is performed using soaked gauzes with Xylocain hydrochloride 5% and naphazoline 0.02% set on the nasal floor and on the medial wall of the inferior turbinate. We have left the infiltration of the turbinate and given the possible neurovegetative complications described by Ravikumar et al. [20].

This procedure is performed under the endoscopic guidance using an 0° endoscope 4-mm diameter. The microdebrider is a device that consist of a handpiece on which is positioned a rotating blade protected by a blunt end that sucks and removes the hypertrophic tissue. The surgeon moves the blade of the microdebrider, with 2300–3000 rev/s speed of oscillation, along the inferior turbinate from posterior to anterior region and with continuous suction. It is suggested to proceed in posteroanterior direction to obtain a clean field, free of blood. The timing of surgery necessary to accomplish the procedure is about 1–2 min long for each nasal cavity [3, 20]. At the end of the surgery, nasal packing of variable length between 8 and 10 cm are placed.

Nasal packing are used to prevent postoperative bleeding and to fill the dead space inside the nasal cavity [21], where it remains only for 48 h and does not change the functional recovery of the mucosa [3]. The patient is advised to instill nasal drops containing vitamin A and Vaseline oil for about a month after surgery [3].

Microdebrider technique is mainly discussed because of its supposed interference on mucociliary clearance.

According to Lee and Lee [21], the microdebrider causes minimal mucosal damage that does not significantly modify the ciliary mucus transport time. In fact, the entire respiratory epithelium of the nasal cavities, and not only the mucosa of the inferior turbinate, is responsible for this physiological mechanism.

According to a study conducted by our University Clinic in the 2012, the microdebrider does not damage the respiratory epithelium, but rather stimulated its regeneration. Studies conducted on animal models have shown that basal cells move the bare mucosa forward after a mechanical injury. The cells undergo transient squamous metaplasia, and then they differentiate both goblet and ciliated cells. This mechanism has also been demonstrated in human nasal cavities. The debridement of the mucosa leads to an improvement in nasal obstruction, rhinorrhea, hyposmia, headaches, snoring, and postnasal drip. It is never associated with consequences such as dryness, crusts, or nasal irritation or with alteration of mucosal function [3].

According to a study conducted by Van et al. [22], the use of the microdebrider technique allowed a success of 93% and only 17 patients presented temporary complications such as bleeding, crusting, and synechia [21]. Lee and Lee have demonstrated, through a 2006 study, that the use of the microdebrider is more effective than the group of patients who have been treated with coblation in obstructive symptomatology and in reducing the volume of the mucosa of the head of the inferior turbinate 12 months after the intervention [21]. It has been defined as the best technique for the treatment of inferior turbinates hypertrophy [3].

2.2 Superficial extramucosal procedures

Superficial extramucosal procedures include

1. Laser-assisted ablation

2. Electrocautery

3. Chemosurgery

4. Cryoturbinectomy

5. Argon plasma coagulation

6. Infrared coagulation

2.2.1 Laser-assisted ablation

Argon laser has been the first application of laser surgery for inferior turbinate, and has been performed by Lenz et al. in 1977 [23], even if was popularized only in the 1990s [24].

Laser surgery has been described with many different procedures such as interstitial, contact, or noncontact. This technique has been performed in topical anesthesia, with slow risk of bleeding, with high compliance of patient.

Many types of lasers have been used for turbinate reduction. They differ in wavelength: CO_2 (λ: 10,600 nm), diode (λ: 940 nm), Ho:YAG laser (λ: 2080 nm), Nd:YAG laser (λ: 1064 nm), argon-ion (λ: 488–514 nm), and potassium-titanyl-phosphate (KTP) with a wavelength similar to Argon laser [25].

The CO_2 laser, Nd:YAG laser, and diode laser has been the light source most used [10] in surgery. Pulsed light mode has been safer than continuous light mode with lesser local damage.

The application of light can be straight as longitudinal strip (laser-strip carbonization) with cross-light beams (cross hatched) and in "single-spots" at a range of 1–2 mm. The most used is the laser strip carbonization. Many studies showed that the best use of this kind of laser for the turbinate is "single-spots," because to be able to preserve healthy portions of mucous for the rapid epithelization [26].

The CO_2 laser has a high cutting precision and superficial vaporization, but is not more maneuverable; above all, for the posterior section of the inferior turbinate, indeed it does not have a flexible optical fiber. CO_2 laser has worse capacity of coagulation, higher price, and worse handling than Ho:YAG, argon-ion, Nd:YAG, and KTP lasers.

Diode laser has been used for the turbinate surgery because it has a good capacity of coagulation of soft tissue with minimal risk to damage the periosteum [27].

YAG laser has a good capacity of penetration of deep tissue respecting the superficial epithelium with a good intraoperative hemostasis but in literature has been reported the presence of post operatory edema with an initial respiratory obstruction, for this reason its use has greatly reduced over time [28].

Potassium titanyl phosphate (KTP) laser is an efficient method to treat a tissue with a high vascularity, as the inferior turbinate had a wavelength that is selectively absorbed by endogenous chromophore as melanin and hemoglobin [29]. In this way, it has a selective action toward submucosal tissue, sparing surface mucosa. Tissue sample treated with KTP surgery is evaluated macroscopically and histologically: necrotizing sialometaplasia, cartilage destruction, and dilated glands with excess mucus occurred, whereas cilia were present [30].

Many authors agree that laser surgery produces permanent histologic changes in turbinate soft tissue [31]: reduction of gland serum mucous and damage of the superficial epithelium with reduction of mucociliary transport [32]. All these change have implications for the postoperative period with presence of scabs and dry mucous. Despite its first listed disadvantages, CO_2 laser is the least damaging of all lasers [33].

2.2.2 Electrocautery

This method uses the heat to clot the soft tissue, causing necrosis and fibrosis with volume reduction of the turbinate. The risk of intra- and postoperative bleeding is uncommon, but the presence of scab and scarring is frequent. Due to the high temperature achieved, this technique is destructive on the mucous and can reduce the efficiency of mucociliary transport [34]. The electrocautery exist in two modalities: monopolar and bipolar. The use of bipolar mode is safer and more effective for significant nasal obstruction reduction [35].

2.2.3 Chemosurgery

In 1926, Denker and Kahler described the use of trichloroacetic acid [36] (TCA) solution to the inferior turbinate in the hypertrophic rhinitis. The effect of TCA consists in protein degeneration [37]. This action on turbinate mucosa is aggressive and damages the mucociliary function. We can study the mucociliary function with the "saccharine time" (ST) [36]: when a saccharine granule is adhered to the nasal mucosa it is dissolved within 1 min, the molecules are then transported to the nasopharynx where the patient recognizes the sweet taste, if the ST is short there is an efficient mucociliary function. In 2008, many authors showed that the "saccharine time" (ST) has been reduced in the early and late period after the TCA application. TCA treatment can induce inhibition of Th2 cell infiltration, a condition typical of allergic rhinitis [38].

2.2.4 *Cryoturbinectomy*

This method is characterized by an application on the surface of inferior turbinate of nitrous oxide for a period of 90–120 s at the −40/−80°C. The cryotherapy causes the formation intracellular of ice crystals and the demolition of cell membrane [39]. A recent paper suggests that regeneration of healthy ciliated nasal epithelium is a constant feature without evidence of scarring [40]. The efficacy on vasomotor rhinitis has been showed [39], but is not sustainable overtime [41].

2.2.5 *Argon plasma coagulation*

Argon plasma coagulation (APC) originally has been used on gastrointestinal lesions under endoscopy then it has been introduced into otolaryngological field [42]. In this method, the current flow is conducted through ionized argon gas (so-called plasma) [43]. The equipment consists of a deliverer of argon gas connected to a high-frequency current generator; the argon, ionized by the monopolar current, covers the surface of the area to be coagulated, without touching it, with a penetration inside the tissue of not more than 2–3 mm [44]. The short tissue vaporization, the rapid application, and the very short propagation of postcoagulation smoke bring further advantages in the performance of small operations in restricted areas as into nasal region [45].

2.2.6 *Infrared coagulation*

Infrared coagulation (IC) has been performed for the first time in 1975 by Nath and Kiefhaber [45]. The light reflects from a 15-V tungsten-halogen lamp from a gold surface. The reflected light has been a spectral maximum in the infrared range: 10,000 A. The tip causes a thermal necrosis on the tissue at 100°C without surface adhesion or carbonization [46]. IC of inferior turbinate seems to be easy to use and safe. It has low cost and patient acceptance. These features make it an attractive alternative to other methods currently used for turbinate reduction [46]. However, the efficacy of this method is especially on the head of inferior turbinate, because the tip is bulky and has an angle of 30° with their column and is hard to perform on the posterior portion of the turbinate [46].

2.3 Turbinate dislocation techniques

Turbinate dislocation techniques include:

1. Inferior turbinate lateralization (or outfracture)

2. Conchopexy

2.3.1 Inferior turbinate lateralization

The inferior turbinate lateralization is a routinely performed procedure. It is a simple technique introduced by Killian in 1904 in order to avoid turbinectomy complications [34, 47]. It is usually performed by using a Goldman or a Freer elevator or a long nosed nasal speculum. The procedure usually begins with an infracture of the inferior turbinate bone (the inferior aspect of the turbinate is pulled medially). An external force is then applied to the turbinate leading to a bone fracture and a dislocation of the turbinate to the lateral nasal wall (**Figure 5**) [48]. This procedure does not modify the anatomy of the surrounding structures, dislocate the uncinate process [49], and close the Hassner valve; hence, there is no blockage of lacrimal duct.

However, the outfracture provides only a temporary improvement of nasal respiration, because the dislocated turbinate often resumes its original position [50]. Generally, this procedure is associated with septoplasty or rhinoplasty. It is also associated with other turbinate reduction techniques because it does not treat the hypertrophy of the turbinate. It is particularly indicated in cases of bony hypertrophy. In order to perform this procedure, it is necessary that the inferior meatus is sufficiently large to contain the dislocated turbinate [51].

In 1990, O'Flynn et al. invented the "multiple submucosal outfracture" (**Figure 6**) in order to improve the efficacy of the outfracture procedure: a little incision is practiced at the cephalic portion of the turbinate near the turbinate bone; the mucosa and the submucosa are elevated with a periosteal elevator and the turbinal bone is fractured into six to eight portions and the bony fragments are dislocated laterally [52].

2.3.2 Conchopexy or concho-antropexy

It was described for the first time by Fateen in 1967. It consisted in a dislocation of the inferior turbinate into the maxillary sinus after antrostomy or demolition of part of the lateral nasal wall [53]. Although the efficacy of this technique had no success, it is now considered obsolete.

2.4 Submucosal procedures

Submucosal procedures include:

1. Submucous resection (or turbinectomy)
2. Cold technique turbinoplasty
    i. With manual instrumentation
    ii. With electronic tools
3. Thermal turbinoplasty
    i. Diatermocoagulation
    ii. Laser surgery
    iii. Radiofrequency (RFAIT)
    iv. Radiofrequency coblation technique (RFCT)

v. Ultrasound

vi. Quantic molecular resonance

vii. Submucosal corticosteroids injection

2.4.1 Submucous resection

Submucous resection was first described by Spielberg in 1924 [54] and then elaborated by Howard House in 1951 [32]. It consists of removing the inferior turbinal bone and the submucosal erectile tissue with preservation of the overlying mucosa [55]. A premedication with vasoconstrictors and local anesthetics is used for both the medial and lateral surfaces of the turbinal mucosa. The Freer knife is used to perform incision over the head of turbinate and is inserted to the previously exposed anterior edge of the conchal bone. The mucosa is separated from the bone by repeated small cutting strokes. The mucoperiosteum is separated from the medial and the lateral surfaces of the bone for a distance of 1.5 cm. The thick

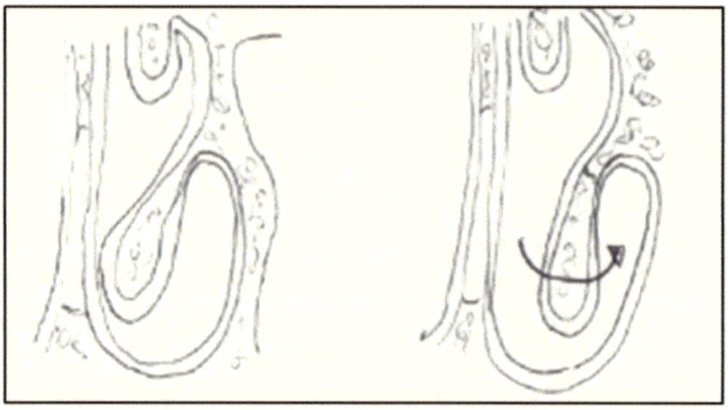

Figure 5.
Inferior turbinate outfracture.

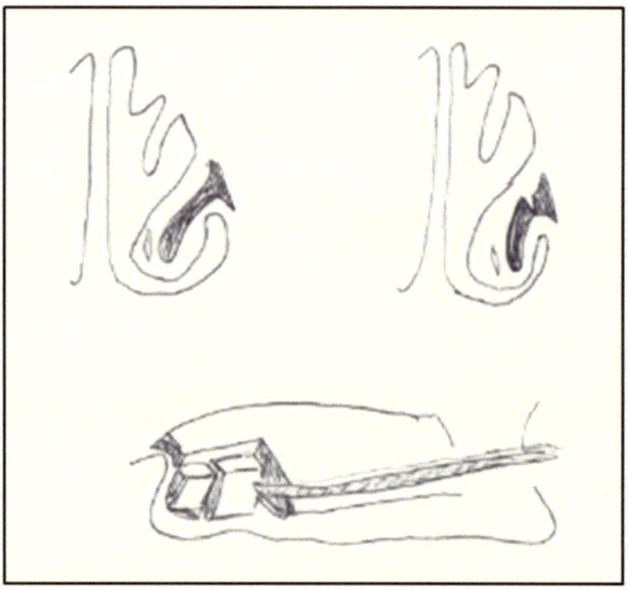

Figure 6.
Multiple submucosal outfracture.

anterior portion of the turbinal bone is grasped with the Takahashi forceps, rotated and then removed. The remaining 2/3 of the bones are very thin, so there is no need to remove it. Sutures are not necessary [32]. By maintaining the mucosal flaps, the normal nasal function is preserved. There is a minimum risk for crusts formation, except for the incision site. There is a low risk for postoperative bleeding, but postoperatively nasal packing is necessary. This technique is particularly effective in cases of prominent bony hypertrophy. A mucosal shredding in inexperienced hands may occur [55]. The submucosal resection leads to fibrosis of the submucosal tissue from the deep layers of the turbinate with the reduction of the immunocompetent cells and IgE. The resection also provokes a damage of the postnasal nerve fibers resulting in the reduction of sneezing and rhinorrhea in allergic patients [56, 57].

2.4.2 Cold turbinoplasty

2.4.2.1 Cold turbinoplasty with manual instrumentation

Turbinoplasty was first described by Mabry in 1982 (**Figure 7**). According to Mabry's technique, a No. 15 blade is used to make an incision from the inferior tip of the turbinate, down to the level of conchal bone, until the posterior edge of the turbinate. A mucosal flap is prepared and elevated from the medial surface. The inferior and lateral part of the turbinate (including bone, soft tissue and lateral mucosa) are then removed with forceps. The residual mucosal-covered soft tissue flap is then curled upon itself to form a "neoturbinate" [58].

2.4.2.2 Cold turbinoplasty with electronic tools (microdebrider)

Powered microdebrider-assisted turbinoplasty is an effective technique with fewer complications of crusting and similar favorable outcomes to manual submucosal resection [55]. It is performed under endoscopic guidance. Local infiltration is given in the inferior turbinate. A vertical incision is made in the anterior tip of the inferior turbinate. The microdebrider is then introduced through the incision and by rotating continuously in a circular fashion it removes all stromal tissue [59]. Finally, anterior nasal packing is kept in nasal passages for 48 h [1]. Microdebrider offers preservation of both the mucosa and the anatomy/physiology of the turbinate. However, this technique is associated with a major risk of postoperative bleeding [55].

2.4.3 Thermal turbinoplasty

2.4.3.1 Submucosal electrocauterization (Diathermy)

This technique was first introduced by Beck in 1930. It is performed using an Abbey needle at 20 W of power. Under endoscopic guidance, the needle is introduced in the anterior tip of the inferior turbinate until the posterior edge. A second pass is performed along the inferior medial edge and a third pass midway between the previous passes. This technique is associated with more complications, such as postoperative bleeding, crusts formation, mucosal dryness, edema, and avascular necrosis [60, 61].

2.4.3.2 Laser surgery

Laser treatment of the inferior turbinates is generally used as extra mucosal technique. Potassium-titanyl-phosphate (KTP) laser has been applied directly inside the turbinate to reduce the vascular tissue. KPT laser energy is well absorbed by hemoglobin and pigmented tissue. Thus, the engorged vessels strongly absorb

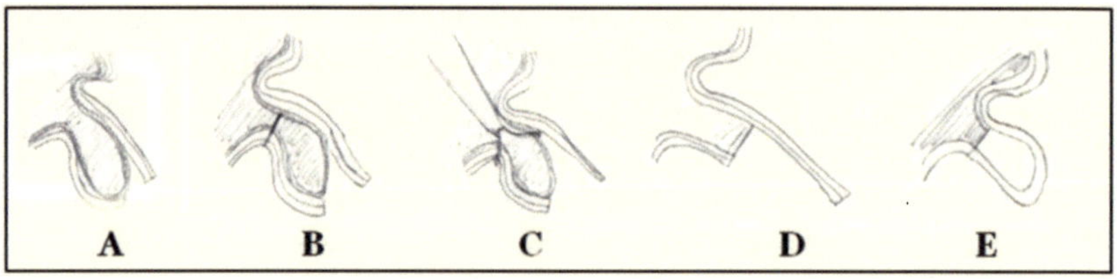

Figure 7.
Cold turbinoplasty with manual instrumentation (Mabry's technique) (A) incision from the inferior tip of the turbinate, (B) mucosal flap, (C and D) the bone and soft tissue of the inferior and lateral part of the turbinate lateral mucosa removal. (E) Residual mucosal curled upon itself to form a "neoturbinate."

the laser energy resulting in shrinkage of the vessels and submucosal tissue. The procedure is conducted as described: an 18-gauge needle is inserted into the submucosa of the inferior turbinate from its anterior edge to about 2 cm. KTP laser is delivered by inserting the fiber through lumen of the needle previously applied, the needle is removed and a retrograde photocoagulation is performed. Results seem to be good with the respect of the mucosa. Patients complain about the long period they have to wait for healing [62, 63].

2.4.3.3 Radiofrequency ablation of the inferior turbinate (RFAIT)

Among the thermal techniques, radiofrequency ablation of the inferior turbinate is one the most performed because of its simple utilization, the possibility to be performed even only under local anesthesia, and its rare complications [64, 65].

This method works generating a high frequency, but low intensity energy. The instrument consists of a monopolar or bipolar generator and a handpiece (probe) that contains electrodes [66]. The electrodes do not get heated themselves [67]. They induce an ionic stirring, and collision between ions and tissue molecules gives out heat over the surrounding submucosal layer of the turbinates (2–4 mm around the active portion of the electrode), preserving overlying mucosal integrity within its mucociliary function. The temperature achieved is always controlled (60–90°C) and carbonization phenomena are excluded [68].

The tip of the electrodes can be introduced in front part (or "head") of the inferior turbinate in one time and pushed across all its length (single insertion site technique) or in three steps (head, body, tail of turbinate), ideally under endoscopic guide. Some authors usually manage just the anterior hypertrophy of the turbinate, as responsible of most nasal resistances [69].

The reduction of the volume of the turbinate is visible just during the surgery, but long term results cannot be estimated during the procedure.

In the first 24–48 h, nasal obstruction can get worse because of the edematous reaction [69], to improve in the following 2–3 weeks, in which the original tissue is replaced by scar tissue, which has a lower thickness. The shrinkage of turbinates enhances with the partial subsequent reabsorption of the scar tissue and the submucosal fibrosis [68] that join the mucosa to the periosteum of the inferior nasal concha. Blood flow is reduced too. Intraoperative and postoperative complications (such as hemorrhage) are rare, and usually there is no need in nasal cavity packing [68].

This surgical option is repeatable and its repetition can stabilize results over time [68].

2.4.3.4 Radiofrequency coblation technique

A different type of radiofrequency bipolar technique is the so-called coblation (term that derives from the union of the words "Cold" and "Ablation") that consists of a bipolar wand and a standard electrosurgical unit. The thermal lesion of the submucosal tissue is caused by the ionic agitation of an electrically conductive fluid (normal saline) added in the space between the electrode and the tissue. This ionic agitation determines a molecular disintegration that is minimal because of the minimum distance between the active and passive electrodes. For the turbinate surgery, two probes are available: the "Reflex Ultra 45 wand" and the "Hummingbird wand" [70, 71].

The surgeon, using the wand, under optical guidance, can create a tissue channel or more, depending on the size of the inferior turbinate to be reduced. In this technique, which can be conducted even under local anesthesia, the infiltration of the turbinate with saline solution is important. Radiofrequency energy promotes a submucosal fibrosis process, which leads to the dimensional reduction of the turbinate, in the absence of involvement of the mucosal lining and/or of the mucociliary transport system. Nasal packing is not required [70].

In the short-term postoperative period, often it is usual to observe a "rebound swelling" of the turbinate, due to the tissue edema, that can last even 10 days, to resolve its self in about 6 weeks. As the common radiofrequency technique or even more frequently, additional therapeutic sessions can be necessary, because of a gradual recurrence of symptoms after some time. Patients with the lowest preoperative nasal conductance of airflow gain greatest objective benefit from turbinate coblation. This means that patient selection with objective measurements is very important [72].

2.4.3.5 Ultrasound

The mechanism of action of this technique consists of the transformation of low frequency ultrasounds (44 + 4.4 KHz) into mechanical oscillations, induced by an acoustic transducer, through a piezoelectric phenomenon. The probe, introduced into the turbinate submucosa through the creation of two parallel intraparenchymal tunnels, ultimately produces a process of ultrasonic disintegration, particularly evident at the level of the cavernous and connective tissue, with reduction of the volume of the turbinate due to the formation of abundant intramural fibrotic tissue. A histopathological analysis with an electronic microscope showed regeneration of respiratory epithelium (ciliary regeneration), after 3 months reduction of hyperplasia; decrease in the number of goblet cells and glandular elements; and restoration of a normal pseudo-layered ciliated epithelium, after 6 months [73, 74].

2.4.3.6 Molecular quantum resonance (QMR)

Unlike the other existing technologies, which base their operating principle on a transfer of thermal energy (heat generated by the passage of current), the molecular quantum resonance scalpel suitably modulated to produce tissue separation not by thermal vaporization, but as a consequence of the "resonance" effect at the cellular level. The energetic quanta, opportunely calibrated for the tissue to be treated, are able to break the molecular bonds inside the cell, without increasing the kinetic energy and, therefore, without increasing the temperature. The result is an extremely precise and delicate biological result, in the absence of damage necrosis. The temperature reached does not exceed 45°C. For the coagulation process, the frequencies are slightly modified, so as to make the molecules vibrate inside the cell and induce a modest rise in temperature (up to about 63°C), which in turn allows to obtain the coagulation of the tissue affected by fibrinogen protein decline. Submucosal decongestion of the turbinate is performed by means of insertion with a headpiece, activated by a QMR machine, so-called Quantum (Telea, Sandrigo-Vicenza, Italy), for a total of 20–30 s, at an intensity force of 3.5, with immediate causes a shrinkage of the mucosa. Since this is a substantially new technique, even if a special dedicated bipolar electrode exists and it is already operating regularly, there are only a few references in the current literature [6, 75].

2.4.3.7 Submucosal corticosteroids injection

The injection of a "long acting" steroid solution is a minimally invasive method, which still guarantees a rather limited benefit over time (it is maximum after 1 week and generally lasts for no longer than a month). It is performed by a slow submucosal injection of triamcinolone acetonide at the level of the turbinate head. A possible complication, even if extremely rare, consists of a transient or permanent loss of sight, which is thought to derive from a retinal vasospasm or a retrograde embolization affecting the retinal circulation (devastating retinal thromboses can also occur) [6, 76, 77].

3. Conclusions

The great interest in turbinate surgery is documented by the large number of surgical techniques proposed over the years and by the production of specific surgical devices by the healthcare industry. However, this diversity of opinions and the quantity of proposed techniques, all valid and scientifically documented, underlines the continuous research to balance the need to solve the obstruction and to maintain the function of the nasal mucosa that unfortunately, in chronic pathologies, like vasomotor rhinitis, is still severely damaged. In literature, in fact, a reduction in epithelial thickness and disappearance of ciliated and goblet cells, the absence of tight junctions, nasal mucus overproduction, inflammatory infiltration in lamina propria [73], marked disruption of the intercellular spaces, and frequent basement membrane interruption [78] can be observed. The lack of mucociliary clearance, absence of tight junctions, widening of intercellular spaces, and discontinuity of the basement membrane induce a reduction in epithelial defense functions, so that environmental factors may directly act on subepithelial structures. As a result, in the nasal respiratory mucosa, an increased responsiveness of trigeminal afferent fibers and secretory and vascular reflexes might occur representing the basis of symptoms [79].

The presence of these profound alterations makes us understand that a preservation of histologically altered mucosa translates inevitably into maintaining an impaired nasal function. On the other hand, it was to demonstrate [2] that the total removal of the nasal mucosa with "cold technique," without high temperatures, that burned and damaged the edges of the removed mucosa, results in a subsequent complete ultrastructural restoration of the healthy tissue.

For this reason, any technique, among those described, the surgeon want to adopt, in any case will have to follow any simple rules: do not use high temperatures, do not remove bone tissue and remove all the hypertrophic and damaged mucosa.

Acknowledgements

I have to thank Dr. Fiorella Cazzato who, with skill and ability, illustrated the present work by enriching it with the original explanatory drawings of various techniques.

Conflict of interest

The authors declare that there is no conflict of interest regarding the publication of this article. All authors have seen and approved the manuscript being submitted. We warrant that this chapter is the authors' original work. We warrant that the chapter has not received prior publication and is not under consideration for publication elsewhere. This research has not been submitted for publication nor has it been published in whole or in part elsewhere. We attest to the fact that all authors listed on the title page have contributed significantly to the work, have read the manuscript, attested to the validity and legitimacy of the data and its interpretation, and agreed to its submission.

Author details

Giampiero Neri[1*], Fiorella Cazzato[1], Elisa Vestrini[1], Pasquina La Torre[1], Giampaolo Quaternato[1], Letizia Neri[1] and Lucia Centurione[2]

1 Neurosciences, Imaging and Clinical Sciences Department, University "G. d'Annunzio", Chieti-Pescara, Italy

2 Medicine and Aging Sciences Department, Section of Human Morphology, University "G. d'Annunzio", Chieti-Pescara, Italy

*Address all correspondence to: neri@unich.it

References

[1] Romano A, Dell'Aversana Orabona G, Salzano G, Abbate V, Iaconetta G, Califano L. Comparative study between partial inferior turbinectomy and microdebrider-assisted inferior turbinoplasty. The Journal of Craniofacial Surgery. 2015;**26**(3):235-238

[2] Neri G, Cazzato F, Mastronardi V, Pugliese M, Centurione MA, Di Pietro R, et al. Ultrastructural regenerating features of nasal mucosa following microdebrider- assisted turbinoplasty are related to clinical recovery. Journal of Translational Medicine. 2016;**14**:164-170

[3] Neri G, Mastronardi V, Traini T, D'Orazio F, Pugliese M, Cazzato F. Respecting nasal mucosa during turbinate surgery: End of the dogma? Rhinology. 2013;**51**(4):368-375

[4] Berger G, Balum-Azim M, Ophir D. The normal inferior turbinate: histomorphometric analysis and clinical implications. Laryngoscope. 2003;**113**(7):1192-1198

[5] Anderson M, Liang J. Trends in inferior turbinate surgery: Analysis of patients using the Medicare database. International Forum of Allergy & Rhinology. 2018;**8**(10):1169-1174

[6] Pagella F, Pusateri A, Danè G, et al. Indicazioni alla chirurgia riduttiva dei turbinati inferiori e work-up preoperatorio acta. In: XXXIV National Congress AOOI; 14-15 October 2010. Verona, Italy; 2010. pp. 207-208

[7] Ferrario F. La chirurgia riduttiva dei turbinati inferiori: Classificazione, rassegna analitica e criteri di selezione degli interventi. In: Acta XXXIV National Congress AOOI; 14-15 October 2010. Verona, Italy; 2010. pp. 213-268

[8] Jones AS, Lancer JM. Does submucosal diathermy to the inferior turbinate reduce nasal resistance to airflow in the long term? The Journal of Laryngology and Otology. 1987;**101**(5):448-451

[9] Talmon Y, Samet A, Gilbey P. Total inferior turbinectomy: Operative results and technique. The Annals of Otology, Rhinology, and Laryngology. 2000;**109**(12):1117-1119

[10] Tasca I, Ceroni Compadretti G, Sorace F, Bacciu A. La chirurgia dei turbinati. In: Tasca I, Manzini M, editors. La chirurgia funzionale del naso. Quaderni Monografici di Aggiornamento A.O.O.I. Galatina, Italy: TorGraf; 2006. p. 85

[11] Huizing EH, deGroot JA. Nasal Pyramid Surgery. In: Huizing EH, de Groot JA, editors. Functional Reconstructive Nasal Surgery. Rome, Italy: Verduci Editore. 2006. p. 278

[12] Garth RJ, Cox HJ, Thomas MR. Haemorrhage as a complication of inferior turbinectomy: A comparison of anterior and radical trimming. Clinical Otolaryngology and Allied Sciences. 1995;**20**(3):236-238

[13] Chevretton EB, Hopkins C, Black IM, Tierney P, Smeeton NC. Degloving of the inferior turbinates: Pilot study to assess the effectiveness of a new technique in turbinate reduction. The Journal of Laryngology and Otology. 2003;**117**(11):866-870

[14] Huizing EH. Functional surgery in inflammation of the nose and paranasal sinuses. Rhinology - Supplement. 1988;**5**:5-15

[15] Kumar D, Rajashekar M. Comparative study of improvement of nasal symptoms following septoplasty with partial inferior turbinectomy

versus septoplasty alone in adults by NOSE Scale: A prospective study. Indian Journal of Otolaryngology and Head & Neck Surgery. 2016;**68**(3):275-284

[16] Passali D, Bellussi L, Damiani V, et al. Allergic rhinitis in Italy: Epidemiology and definition of most commonly used diagnostic and therapeutic modalities. Acta Otorhinolaryngologica Italica. 2003;**23**:257-264

[17] Sapçi T, Sahin B, Karavus A, Akbulut UG. Comparison of the effects of radiofrequency tissue ablation, CO_2 laser ablation, and partial turbinectomy applications on nasal mucociliary functions. The Laryngoscope. 2003;**113**(3):514-519

[18] Salzano FA, Mora R, Dellepiane M, et al. Radiofrequency, high-frequency, and electrocautery treatments vs partial inferior turbinotomy: Microscopic and macroscopic effects on nasal mucosa. Archives of Otolaryngology – Head & Neck Surgery. 2009;**135**(8):752-758

[19] Davis WE, Nishioka GJ. Endoscopic partial inferior turbinectomy using a power microcutting instrument. Ear, Nose, & Throat Journal. 1996;**75**(1):49-50

[20] Ravikumar A, Griffith TD, Flood LM, McNeela BJ. An unusual complication following inferior turbinectomy. The Journal of Laryngology and Otology. 1995;**109**(6):559-561

[21] Lee JY, Lee JD. Comparative study on the long-term effectiveness between coblation- and microdebrider-assisted partial turbinoplasty. The Laryngoscope. 2006;**116**(5):729-734

[22] Van delden MR, Cook PR, Davis WE. Endoscopic partial inferior turbinoplasty. Otolaryngology and Head and Neck Surgery. 1999;**121**(4):406-409

[23] Lenz H, Eichler J, Schafer G, Salk J. Parameters for argon-laser surgery of the lower human turbinates. Acta Oto-Laryngologica. 1977;**83**(3-4):360-365

[24] Bergmark RW, Gray ST. Surgical management of turbinate hypertrophy. Otolaryngologic Clinics of North America. 2018;**51**(5):919-928

[25] Freer OT. The inferior turbinate: Its longitudinal resection for chronic intumescence. Laryngoscope. 1911;**21**:1136-1144

[26] Lippert BM, Werner JA. Comparison of carbon dioxide and neodymium: Yttrium-aluminum-garnet lasers in surgery of the inferior turbinate. The Annals of Otology, Rhinology, and Laryngology. 1997;**106**(12):1036-1042

[27] Janda P, Sroka R, Tauber S, Baugartner R, Grevers G, Leunig A. Diode laser treatment of hyperplastic inferior nasal turbinates. Lasers in Surgery and Medicine. 2000;**27**(2):129-139

[28] Metson R. Holmium:YAG laser endoscopic sinus surgery: A randomized, controlled study. The Laryngoscope. 1996;**106**(Suppl. 77):1-18

[29] Wang HK, Tsai YH, Wu YY, Wang PC. Endoscopic potassium-titanyl-phosphate laser treatment for the reduction of hypertrophic inferior nasal turbinate. Photomedicine and Laser Surgery. 2004;**22**(3):173-176

[30] Somogyvári K, Móricz P, Gerlinger I, Kereskai L, Szanyi I, Takács I. Morphological and histological effects of radiofrequency and laser (KTP and Nd:YAG) treatment of the inferior turbinates in animals. Surgical Innovation. 2017;**24**(1):5-14

[31] Wexler DB, Berger G, Derowe A, Ophir D. Long-term histologic effects of inferior turbinate laser surgery.

Otolaryngology and Head and Neck Surgery. 2001;**124**(4):459-463

[32] House HP. Submucous resection of the inferior turbinal bone. Laryngoscope. 1951;**61**(7):637-648

[33] Martinez SA, Nissen AJ, Stock CR, Tesmer T. Nasal turbinate resection for relief of nasal obstruction. Laryngoscope. 1983;**93**(7):871-875

[34] Hol MKS, Huizing EH. Treatment of inferior turbinate pathology: A review and critical evaluation of the different techniques. Rhinology. 2000;**38**(4):157-166

[35] Rao SUP, Basavaraj P, Yempalle SB, Ramachandra AD. A prospective study of different methods of inferior turbinate reduction. Journal of Clinical and Diagnostic Research. 2017;**11**(5):MC01-MC03

[36] Sakakura Y, Ukai K, Majima Y, Murai S, Harada T, Miyoshi Y. Nasal mucociliary clearance under various conditions. Acta Oto-Laryngologica. 1983;**96**(1-2):167-173

[37] Unsal Tuna EE, Ozbek C, Koç C, Ozdem C. Evaluation of nasal symptoms and mucociliary function in patients with allergic rhinitis treated with chemosurgery using trichloroacetic acid. American Journal of Otolaryngology. 2008;**29**(1):37-41. DOI: 10.1016/j.amjoto.2006.12.006

[38] Yao K, Sato K, Usui D, Kurihara R, Okamoto M, Iguchi Y, et al. Chemosurgery with trichloroacetic acid for allergic rhinitis: Evaluation of the efficacy in terms of inhibition of Th2 cell infiltration. Auris, Nasus, Larynx. 2009;**36**(3):292-299

[39] Bumstead RM. Cryotherapy for chronic vasomotor rhinitis: Technique and patient selection for improved results. The Laryngoscope. 1984;**94**(4):539-544

[40] Principato JJ. Chronic vasomotor rhinitis: Cryogenic and other surgical modes of treatment. The Laryngoscope. 1979;**89**(4):619-638

[41] Rakover Y, Rosen G. A comparison of partial inferior turbinectomy and cryosurgery for hypertrophic inferior turbinates. The Journal of Laryngology and Otology. 1996;**110**(8):732-735

[42] Ferri E, Armato E, Cavaleri S, Capuzzo P, Ianniello F. Argon plasma surgery for treatment of inferior turbinate hypertrophy: A long-term follow-up in 157 patients. ORL: Journal for Otorhinolaryngology and Its Related Specialties. 2003;**65**(4):206-210

[43] Scheithauer MO. Surgery of the turbinates and "empty nose" syndrome. GMS Current Topics in Otorhinolaryngology - Head and Neck Surgery. 2010;**9**:1-28

[44] Farin G, Grund KE. Technology of argon plasma coagulation with particle regard to endoscopic application. Endoscopic Surgery and Allied Technologies. 1994;**2**(1):71-77

[45] Nath G. The new principle of infrared coagulation in medicine and its physical fundamentals. Coloproctology. 1981;**3**:379-381

[46] Moulton-Barrett R, Passy V, Horlick D, Brauel G. Infrared coagulation of the inferior turbinate: A new treatment for refractory chronic rhinitis. Otolaryngology and Head and Neck Surgery. 1994;**111**(5):674-679

[47] Salam MA, Wengraf C. Conchoantropexy or total inferior turbinectomy for hypertrophy of the inferior turbinates? A prospective randomized study. The Journal of Laryngology and Otology. 1993;**107**:1125-1128

[48] Jourdy D. Inferior turbinate reduction. Operative Techniques in Otolaryngology. 2014;**25**:160-170

[49] Lee KC, Lee SS, Lee JK, Lee SH. Medial fracturing of the inferior turbinate: Effect on the ostiomeatal unit and the uncinate process. European Archives of Oto-Rhino-Laryngology. 2009;**266**(6):857-861

[50] Goode RL. Surgery of the turbinates. The Journal of Otolaryngology. 1978;7:262-268

[51] Saunders WH. Surgery of the inferior nasal turbinates. The Annals of Otology, Rhinology, and Laryngology. 1982;**91**:445-447

[52] O'Flynn PE, Milford CA, Mackay JS. Multiple submucosal out-fractures of inferior turbinates. The Journal of Laryngology and Otology. 1990;**104**(3):239-240

[53] Fateen M. Concho-antropexy in vasomotor rhinitis and chronic nasal obstruction. Rhinology. 1967;**5**:20-24

[54] Spielberg W. The treatment of nasal obstruction by submucous resection of the inferior turbinate bone. Laryngoscope. 1924;**34**:197-203

[55] Nurse LA, Duncavage JA. Surgery of the inferior and middle turbinate. Otolaryngologic Clinics of North America. 2009;**42**(2):295-309

[56] Mori S, Fujieda S, Yamada T, Limura Y, Takahashi N, Saito H. Long-term effect of submucous turbinectomy in patients with perennial allergic rhinitis. Laryngoscope. 2002;**112**:866-869

[57] El Henawi Del D, Ahmed MR, Madian YT. Comparison between power-assisted turbinoplasty and submucosal resection in the treatment of inferior turbinate hypertrophy. ORL. 2011;**73**(3):151-155

[58] Mabry RL. Inferior turbinoplasty. Laryngoscope. 1982;**92**:459-461

[59] Bruggers S, Sindwani R. Innovations in microdebrider technology and design. Otolaryngologic Clinics of North America. 2009;**42**:781-787

[60] Beck JC. Pathology and intramural electrocoagulation of inferior turbinate. The Annals of Otology, Rhinology, and Laryngology. 1930;**39**:349-363

[61] Hurd LM. Bipolar electrode for electrocoagulation of the inferior turbinate. Archives of Otolaryngology. 1931;**13**:442

[62] Vijayakumar S, Divakaran S, Parida PK, Gopalakrishnan S. Potassium titanyl phosphate laser turbinate reduction in the management of allergic inferior turbinate hypertrophy: Our experience. Allergy & Rhinology. 2016;**7**(1):29-33

[63] Supiyaphun P, Aramwatanapong P, Kerekhanjanarong V, Sastarasadhit V. KTP laser inferior turbinoplasty: An alternative procedure to treat the nasal obstruction. Auris Nasus Larynx. 2003;**30**:59-64

[64] Means C, Camacho M, Capasso R. Long-term outcomes of radiofrequency ablation of the inferior turbinates. Indian Journal of Otolaryngology and Head & Neck Surgery. 2016;**68**(4):424-428

[65] Rhee CS, Kim DY, Won TB, Lee HJ, Park SW, Kwon TY, et al. Changes of nasal function after temperature-controlled radiofrequency tissue volume reduction for the turbinate. The Laryngoscope. 2001;**111**(1):153-158

[66] Hytönen ML, Bäck LJJ, Malmivaara AV, Roine RP. Radiofrequency thermal ablation for patients with nasal symptoms: A systematic review of effectiveness and complications. European Archives of Oto-Rhino-Laryngology. 2009;**266**:1257-1266

[67] Smith TL, Correa AJ, Kuo T, Reinisch L. Radiofrequency tissue ablation of the inferior turbinates using

a thermocouple feedback electrode. Laryngoscope. 1999;**109**:1760-1765

[68] Elwany S, Gaimaee R, Fattah HA. Radiofrequency bipolar submucosal diathermy of the inferior turbinates. American Journal of Rhinology. 1999;**13**:145-149

[69] Cavaliere M, Mottola G, Iemma M. Comparison of the effectiveness and safety of radiofrequency turbinoplasty and traditional surgical technique in treatment of inferior turbinate hypertrophy. Otolaryngology and Head and Neck Surgery. 2005;**133**(6):972-978

[70] Di Rienzo Businco L, Di Rienzo Businco A, Lauriello M. Comparative study on the effectiveness of Coblation-assisted turbinoplasty in allergic rhinitis. Rhinology. 2010;**48**(2):174-178

[71] Chang CW, Ries WR. Surgical treatment of the inferior turbinate: New techniques. Current Opinion in Otolaryngology & Head and Neck Surgery. 2004;**12**:53-57

[72] Farmer SE, Quine SM, Eccles R. Efficacy of inferior turbinate coblation for treatment of nasal obstruction. The Journal of Laryngology and Otology. 2009;**123**(3):309-314

[73] Gindros G, Kantas I, Balatsouras DG, Kandiloros D, Manthos AK, Kaidoglou A. Mucosal changes in chronic hypertrophic rhinitis after surgical turbinate reduction. European Archives of Oto-Rhino-Laryngology. 2009;**266**:1409-1416

[74] Nousia C, Gouveris H, Giatromanolaki A, Ypsilantis P, Katotomichelakis M, Watelet J-B, et al. Ultrasound submucosal inferior nasal turbinate reduction technique: Histological study of wound healing in a sheep model. Rhinology. 2010;**48**:169-173

[75] Di Rienzo Businco L, Di Rienzo Businco A, Ventura L, Laurino S. Turbinoplasty with quantic molecular resonance in the treatment of persistent moderate-severe allergic rhinitis: Comparative analysis of efficacy. American Journal of Rhinology & Allergy. 2014;**28**(2):164-168

[76] Simmons MW. Intranasal injection of corticosteroids. California Medicine. 1960;**92**:155-158

[77] Simmons MW. Intranasal injection of corticosteroids in nasal disorders: Further observations. Pacific Coast Oto-Ophthalmological Society. 1964;**45**:95-103

[78] Berger G, Gass S, Ophir D. The histopathology of the hypertrophic inferior turbinate. Archives of Otolaryngology – Head & Neck Surgery. 2006;**132**:588-594

[79] Giannessi F, Fattori B, Ursino F, Giambelluca A, Soldani P, Scavuzzo MC, et al. Ultrastructural and ultracytochemical study of the human nasal respiratory epithelium in vasomotor rhinitis. Acta Oto-Laryngologica. 2003;**123**:943-949

Chapter 11

Concurrent Rhinoplasty and Endoscopic Sinus Surgery

Balwant Singh Gendeh

Abstract

Combining rhinoplasty and endoscopic sinus surgery (ESS) was first reported in 1991 by Sheman and Matarasso. Since then, many authors have documented a large series showing the overall efficacy of combining the two procedures. The focus of this manuscript is to document the author's recent experience with combining rhinoplasty and endoscopic sinus surgery and highlight the changes that have occurred during the author's 2-years experience. A retrospective data review was performed on 53 (31 females and 22 men, age range 16–55 years) patients who underwent combined rhinoplasty and ESS between January 2016 and December 2018 at Pantai Hospital Kuala Lumpur by the same surgeon. The mean age was 31.8 years. All patients had severe nasal obstruction with chronic rhinosinusitis and were followed up for a minimum of 6 months post-surgery and underwent ENT workup, which included history, office rigid endoscopy, CT scans of paranasal sinuses and preoperative photography. Initially, the ESS was performed followed by the open rhinoplasty with or without osteotomy. The ESS consisted of middle turbinate reduction [15/53 (28.3%)], maxillary antrostomy [36/53 (67.9%)], ethmoidectomy [38/53 (71.6%)], frontal sinusotomy [7/53 (13.2%)], and sphenoidotomy [9/53 (16.9%)]. Most of the sinus symptoms resolved postoperatively with 47 (88.6%) of 53 patients describing their improvement as significant. Fifty (94.3%) of 53 patients stated that they would recommend the concurrent procedure. The benefits of these advances are illustrated by a review of the literature with good results (functional and cosmetic) and minimal complications.

Keywords: rhinoplasty, open, concurrent, endoscopic sinus surgery, one team approach

1. Introduction

There is an increasing demand for facial plastic surgery with more awareness of the procedure and its outcome. Many patients who seek surgery for their nasal aesthetics also have complaints of nasal obstruction and snoring [1, 2]. Severe gross septal deviations present big surgical challenges for the operating surgeon. The role of functional rhinoplasty in the management of internal nasal valve has been discussed by numerous authors (**Figure 1**).

A complete evaluation of these groups of patients with nasal endoscopy and CT scan of paranasal sinuses will often reveal concurrent chronic rhinosinusitis (CRS).

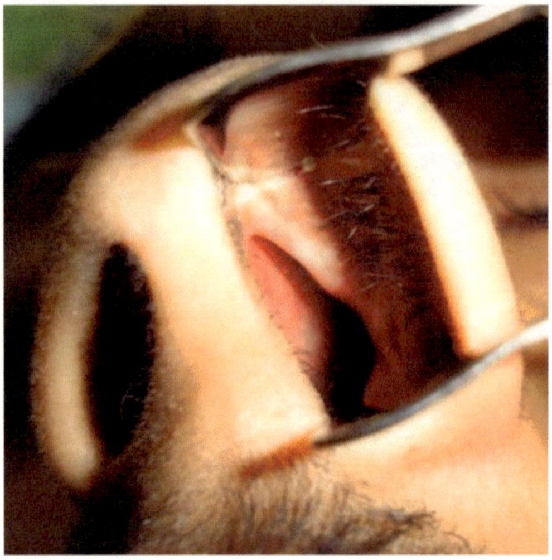

Figure 1.
A close-up view showing the anatomical relationship of the left internal nasal valve to the septum anteromedially and the inferior turbinate laterally.

Procedures of endoscopic sinus surgery (ESS), septoplasty (SP), and rhinoplasty (RP) were initially meant for functional improvement to which today an aesthetic aim is added. The functional aim of rhinoplasty is meant for recovery of normal sinonasal physiology and ventilatory function.

CRS is an inflammation of the nose and paranasal sinuses manifesting with two or more significant symptoms for 12 weeks with endoscopic and/or CT scan signs of disease. The symptoms include nasal obstruction, thick nasal discharge, and/or facial pain/pressure and/or reduction or loss of sense of smell [3]. Diagnosis of CRS is primarily based on symptoms that are confirmed by nasal endoscopy and CT scans in coronal and axial views (**Figures 2** and **3**).

In functional rhinoplasty, the role of the spreader graft [4], columellar extension graft [5], shield graft [6, 7], onlay conchal graft [8], nasal valve suture suspension [9], and flaring sutures [10] has been advocated by numerous authors. Endoscopic sinus surgery (ESS) has also been accepted as a safe and efficient modality for the treatment of CRS. The combination of both these procedures would offer great benefit to the indicated patient group.

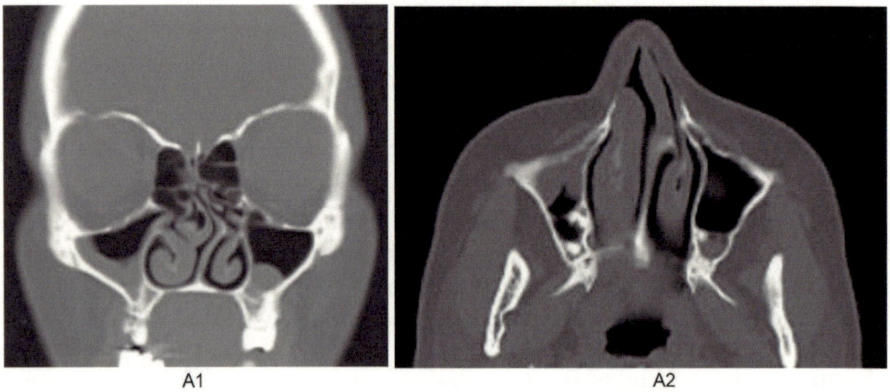

Figure 2.
Coronal (A1) and axial (A2) CT scan serial cuts of paranasal sinuses showing a markedly deviated nasal septum with pneumatized diseased right middle turbinate and evidence of sinusitis.

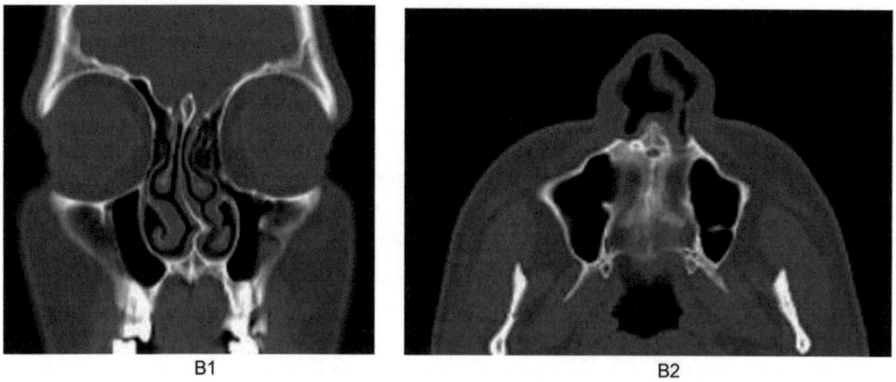

Figure 3.
Coronal (B1) and axial (B2) CT scan serial cuts of paranasal sinuses showing a grossly deviated nasal septum post-trauma with evidence of paranasal sinus mucosal thickening.

Concurrent ESS, SP, and RP are affordable, reliable, and safe procedures when performed as a single surgical procedure to reduce operative time, general anesthetic, and recovery period [11]. The additional RP leads to an increase in postoperative complications but when analyzed separately is considered minor in the literature [12, 13]. Thus, the result of surgery and the patient's quality of life are not exceedingly compromised and therefore considered acceptable. Traditional surgeons have been concerned of combining rhinoplasty and ESS to avoid the possibility of increased postoperative complications. Recent publications have reported initial success with this combined technique [14].

Therefore, a larger sample study like this can better define how RP affects outcomes of concurrent ESS and SP.

We present a novel one surgeon combined endoscopic sinus surgery and rhinoplasty technique to evaluate patient satisfaction, efficacy, safety, and clinical outcomes of them undergoing concurrent surgery.

2. Methods and materials

2.1 Patients

A retrospective clinical chart review was performed on all of the author's patients who had nasal surgery from January 2016 through December 2018 at the ENT unit of Pantai Hospital Kuala Lumpur (PHKL). All patients had severe nasal obstruction with chronic rhinosinusitis and were followed up for a minimum of 6 months post-surgery. The data revealed that 53 patients out of the 116 patients (45.6%) underwent concurrent open rhinoplasty and ESS by the same surgeon at PHKL. Patients who underwent rhinoplasty and ESS at different sittings (54.4%) were excluded from the study because the SNOT 22 subjective scoring system which was used only for the evaluation of patient symptoms in the concurrent group before and after surgery was sufficient, and therefore the need to compare with patients who underwent rhinoplasty and ESS at different sittings was not necessary. A history of nasal trauma and snoring was documented.

Patients with primary nasal dysfunction and sinus complaints were seen by the same surgeon. All the patients underwent ENT workup which included history, head and neck examination, nasal endoscopy, and CT scans of paranasal sinuses and were treated with oral antibiotics and topical nasal steroids prior to the CT scan and a full facial analysis including standardized photography.

2.2 Evaluation

The main complaints of the patients prior to surgery were chronic nasal obstruction, postnasal drip, headaches with occasional voice changes, and snoring. External nasal examination was performed to detect a twisted/crooked/saddled nose.

Nasal endoscopy revealed that all these patients had significant anterior septal deviation involving the internal nasal valve, in addition to posterior septal deviation. Nasal endoscopic examination was performed to detect the grading of septal deviations, namely, I, II, III, IV, and V (**Figure 4**), and diseased mucosal or polypoidal tissue (grade 1, 2, 3) involving the paranasal sinuses. If there was evidence of mucopurulent discharge from the paranasal sinuses on nasal endoscopy on admission, the patients were commenced on systemic antibiotics prior to surgery.

2.3 Surgical technique

All the cases were performed as an inpatient procedure by a one surgeon and two procedure approach under general anesthesia at Pantai Hospital Kuala Lumpur. At the time of induction, all patients received IV antibiotics (ceftriaxone 1 gm) and steroids (dexamethasone 8 mg). The CT scans of the paranasal sinuses were reviewed again in OR prior to performing the surgery. A throat pack was inserted, and the nasal cavity was packed with soaked spacers for vasoconstriction. Infiltration was performed at the nasal dorsum, alar rim, septum, and greater palatine fossa transorally with levobupivacaine (20 cc), adrenaline (0.2 mg), and aqua (1.8 cc). Surgery was initiated with ESS procedure followed by open rhinoplasty approach, but in gross septal deviations, the septoplasty was performed prior to the ESS.

For the open rhinoplasty approach, an inverted transcolumellar V-shaped incision was made, and the SMAS elevated all the way to the dorsum of the nose (**Figure 5**). The domes are divided in the midline, and the upper lateral cartilages released laterally, creating excellent exposure of the septum. Bilateral submucoperichondrial flaps are elevated, exposing the entire cartilaginous and anterior bony septum. The cartilaginous and bony septum is then resected by paramedian

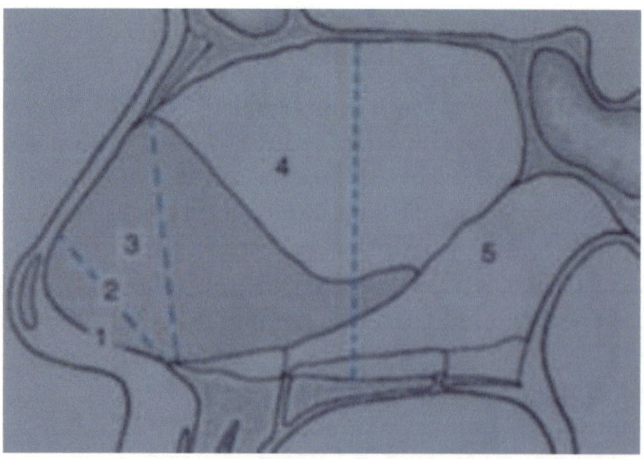

Figure 4.
The five areas of the internal nose most commonly involved in nasal septal deviations. Open approach rhinoplasty is indicated in anterior deviations of nasal septum involving areas I, II, and III along with significant internal nasal valve involvement, whereas closed approach is indicated for posterior septal deviations restricted to areas IV and V only.

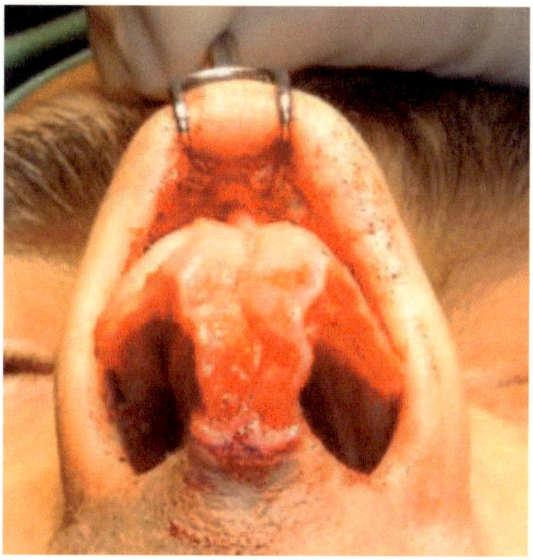

Figure 5.
Close-up view of open rhinoplasty via a transcolumellar incision and elevation of SMAS all the way to the nasal dorsum.

osteotomy, separating cartilaginous septum from maxillary crest and fracturing bony septum as posterior as possible leaving behind the cribriform plate and sphenoid rostrum. Extracorporeal approach was performed on all patients with gross high septal deviation, which requires complete removal of the entire cartilaginous septum, which is then straightened and returned to the nose. In revision rhinoplasty cases where adequate quadrangular cartilage and septal bone grafts were not available, conchal cartilage graft was harvested. Bilateral spreader grafts are then placed on the dorsal part of the septum. K-wire drill was used to drill multiple holes on the septal bone graft for use as spreader/ columella strut/columella extension graft. Straight 4/0 Monosyn mattress sutures were used to secure the spreader graft. Then lateral osteotomies are performed by external subcutaneous method if required. Nasal spine if deviated more than 30° is gauged out or drilled. Neo-septum with spreader graft is inserted in the nose. Areas of fixation are the caudal end of the nasal bones, upper lateral cartilage, and maxillary crest. A hole is drilled through the nasal bones and the nasal spine and suturing the neo-septum with Monosyn 4/0 sutures. Other required steps like columellar strut, rim grafts, and tip grafts are performed. Soft silicon splints are placed along either side of septum and sutured in place with through-and through 3/0 Monosyn sutures. Curve Monosyn 4/0 and 5/0 were used for tip plasty (transcrural, intercrural, shield graft), dorsal augmentation, caudal augmentation, septum augmentation, and alar rim suturing. Ethicon 6/0 sutures were used for the skin.

For the ESS, the mucosa on the lateral wall of the nose and the anterior face of the sphenoid was infiltrated and the diseased sinuses addressed by performing ethmoidectomy, middle meatal antrostomy, sphenoidotomy or frontal sinusotomy. Prior to performing middle meatal antrostomy, an uncinectomy was performed using thru-cut instruments along with a microdebrider.

The nasal and sinus cavities were packed with Nasapore. Steri-Strip was applied externally on the nasal dorsum along with Denver splints which were removed between 7 and 10 days postoperatively. Nasal cavity suction was performed on the third postoperative day along with the removal of the nasal septal splints and patient sent home the same day. The ESS was performed using a technique adapted from Stammberger [12] and Kennedy [13]. The ESS instruments included high-definition Spice monitor, 4 mm endoscopes (0, 30 and 70°), and powered instruments (debrider by Medtronic). IGS was used in revision sinus surgery cases. All patients received postoperative antibiotics and nasal rinse. The one surgeon team performed the postoperative endoscopic debridement and nasal function and documented aesthetic alterations with standardized postoperative photography.

2.4 Data collection

The medical charts of included patients were retrieved for analysis and demographic data obtained (**Table 1**). The medical and surgical history, presenting complaints and physical and endoscopic examination results, was documented. The details of the rhinoplasty and sinus surgery subtype procedures are listed in **Tables 2** and **3**, respectively. Patient follow-ups were obtained with standardized questionnaires (SNOT 22) of presenting complaints, satisfaction with surgical experience, and self-evaluation of aesthetic outcome.

Patient number	Race/country of origin	Age	Sex	Open rhinoplasty (ORP) procedure	ESS procedure	Duration (minutes)	Blood loss (ml)
1	M	34	F	SP, SprG, CEG SG, O	TR, E, MMA	179	95
2	Canada	54	F	SP, SprG, SG	TR	145	115
3	M	39	F	SP, SprG, CEG, SG, O	TR, E, MMA	181	115
4	I	36	M	SP, SprG, SG, HR	TR	148	110
5	I	32	F	SP, SprG, CS, SG	TR, E, MMA	179	90
6*	C	50	F	SP, SprG, CEG SG, O, CCG	TR, E, MMA, FS	287	235
7	C	26	F	SP, SprG, CEG SG	TR	152	80
8	M	30	F	SP, SprG, CEG SG	TR, E, MMA	177	85
9	I	32	F	SP, SprG, SG, CSR	TR, E, MMA, Sph	211	105
10	M	32	M	SP, SprG, CEG SG, O	TR, E, MMA	189	120
11	I	23	F	SP, SprG, SG	TR	141	90
12	Australia	45	F	SP, SprG, SG	TR, E, MMA	185	100
13	I	32	F	SP, SprG, CS, SG	TR, E, MMA	195	95
14	M	18	M	SP, SprG, CEG, SG	TR, E	190	75
15	C	22	F	SP, SprG, CEG, SG	TR, E, MMA	184	110
16	C	40	F	SP, SprG, CEG, SG	TR	164	85
17	M	28	M	SP, SprG, CEG, SG	TR, E, MMA	168	90
18*	M	55	M	SP, SprG, CEG, SG, O	TR, E, MA, FS, Sph, CCG	277	240
19	I	32	F	SP, SprG, SG	TR, E, MMA	171	110
20	M	40	F	SP, SprG, CEG, SG	TR, E, MMA	154	85
21	I	25	M	SP, SprG, CS, SG	TR	159	85
22	I	25	F	SP, SprG, SG	TR	167	105
23	I	29	M	SP, SprG, SG	TR, E, MMA	143	115
24	C	31	F	SP, SprG, CEG, SG	TR, E, MMA	156	95

Patient number	Race/country of origin	Age	Sex	Open rhinoplasty (ORP) procedure	ESS procedure	Duration (minutes)	Blood loss (ml)
25	C	40	F	SP, SprG, CEG, SG	TR, E, MMA	169	105
26	I	25	F	SP, SprG, SG, CSR, O	TR, E, MMA, Sph	191	180
27	United Kingdom	37	M	SP, SprG, SG, O	TR, E, MMA, FS, Sph	261	245
28	M	26	F	SP, SprG, CEG, SG	TR, E, MMA	189	160
29	I	31	M	SP, SprG, CS, SG	TR	148	140
30	C	23	M	SP, SprG, CEG, SG, O	TR, E, MMA, FS	253	215
31	M	25	F	SP, SprG, CEG, SG	TR, E, MMA, Sph	214	120
32	M	36	F	SP, SprG, CEG, SG	TR, E, MMA	197	100
33	I	41	F	SP, SprG, CS, SG	TR	154	80
34	M	25	F	SP, SprG, CEG, SG	TR, E, MMA	176	130
35	I	22	M	SP, SprG, SG	TR, E, MMA, Sph	187	110
36	I	16	M	SP, SprG, SG	TR	160	80
37	C	50	M	SP, SprG, CEG, SG, O	TR, E, MMA	181	105
38*	I	23	M	SP, SprG, CS, SG, O, HR, CCG	TR, E, MMA, FS, Sph	267	210
39	I	33	M	SP, SprG, CEG, SG	TR, E, MMA	191	115
40	Indonesia	38	F	SP, SprG, CEG, SG	TR	169	75
41	I	28	F	SP, SprG, SG, CSR	TR, E, MMA, FS	189	90
42	C	52	F	SP, SprG, CEG, SG	TR, E, MMA	212	95
43	C	30	F	SP, SprG, CEG, SG	TR	172	85
44	I	23	F	SP, SprG, SG, O, HR	TR, E, MA, FS, Sph	265	220
45	I	36	M	SP, SprG, CS, SG	TR	97	110
46	M	41	F	SP, SprG, CEG, SG	TR	163	75
47	C	17	M	SP, SprG, CEG, SG	TR, E, MMA	191	105
48	M	27	M	SP, SprG, CEG, SG, O	TR, E, MMA	183	120
49	Indonesia	32	M	SP, SprG, CEG, SG	TR,E	193	105
50	M	28	M	SP, SprG, CEG, SG	TR, E, MMA	176	115
51	I	18	M	SP, SprG, CS, SG	TR	163	95
52	I	18	F	SP, SprG, CEG, SG, O, HR	TR, E, MMA, FS, Sph	259	250
53	Iran	35	M	SP, SprG, CS, SG	TR, E, MMA	197	120

TR, turbinate reduction; SP, septoplasty; Spr G, spreader graft; CEG, columella extension graft; SG, shield graft; HR, hump reduction; CS, columella strut; CCG, conchal cartilage graft; CSR, caudal septal resection; E, ethmoidectomy; MMA, middle meatal antrostomy; Sph, sphenoidotomy; FS, frontal sinusotomy; M, Malay; C, Chinese; I, Indian *Revision cases*

Table 1.
Demographics of 53 patients who underwent concurrent rhinoplasty and ESS.

Septoplasty (SP)	53 (100%)
Turbinate reduction (TR)	53 (100%)
Ethmoidectomy (E)	38 (71.7%)
Middle meatal antrostomy (MMA)	36 (67.9%)
Sphenoidotomy (Sph)	9 (16.9%)
Frontal sinusotomy (FS)	8 (15.1%)

Table 2.
Summary of endoscopic sinus subtype procedures performed on 53 patients who underwent concurrent two procedural approaches.

Spreader graft (SprG)	53 (100%)
Shield graft (SG)	53 (100%)
Columella extension graft (CEG)	29 (54.7%)
Osteotomy (O)	13 (24.5%)
Columella strut (CS)	9 (16.9%)
Hump reduction (HR)	4 (7.5%)
Caudal septal resection (CSR)	3 (5.6)
Conchal cartilage graft (CCG)	3 (5.6)

Table 3.
Summary of rhinoplasty subtype procedures performed on 53 patients who underwent concurrent two procedural approaches.

3. Results

Between January 2016 and December 2018, 53 patients underwent rhinoplasty combined with endoscopic sinus surgery (ESS). The demography of the patients is listed in **Table 1**. There were 31 females and 22 males with age ranging from 16 to 55 years with a mean of 31.8 years. There were three referred revision cases where rhinoplasty [1] and septoplasty [2] were performed elsewhere. All patients had open approach rhinoplasty. The average operative time was 45 minutes for endoscopic sinus surgery and 141.20 minutes for rhinoplasty. The average operating time for the concurrent procedure was 186.20 minutes, and average blood loss was 121.4 ml. Out of the 53 patients, there were 15 Malays, 11 Chinese, and 21 Indians, and the remaining 6 were foreigners (one each from Australia, Canada, Iran, and the United Kingdom and two from Indonesia). Thirty-eight (71,6%) of the 53 patients had a history of chronic snoring and 27 (50.9%) history of nasal trauma.

Regarding the ESS, the most common procedure performed was septoplasty and turbinate reduction in all patients, followed by ethmoidectomy (71.7%), middle meatal antrostomy (67.9%), sphenoidotomy (16.9%), and frontal sinusotomy (15.1%). Majority of the patients had extensive mucosal disease requiring sinus surgery.

Regarding the rhinoplasty procedures, the most common aesthetic procedure was spreader graft and shield graft in all patients followed by columella extension graft (54.7%), osteotomy (24.5%), columella strut (11.9%), hump reduction (7.5%) caudal septal resection, and conchal cartilage graft (5.6%). It is of interest to note that 53 patients had some type of cartilage graft performed (spreader graft, shield graft, columellar extension graft, caudal septal resection, columella strut, and conchal cartilage graft). Pictures of spreader and shield grafts are illustrated in **Figures 6** and 7. All patients were followed up for a minimum of 6 months of post-surgery at the time of this report. All patients reported an improvement in

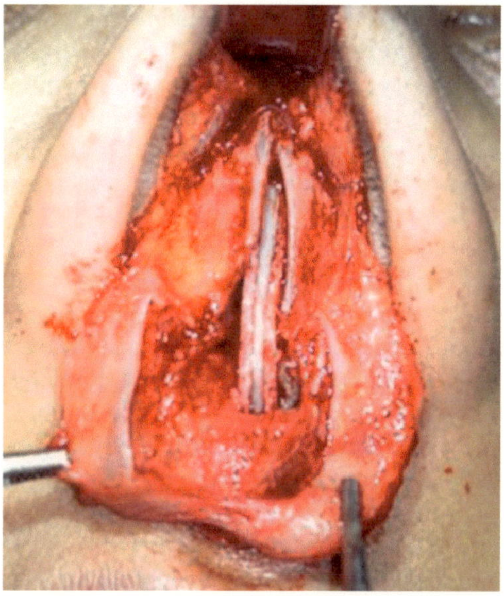

Figure 6.
Picture showing spreader graft sandwiched between the septum just before mattress sutures are applied in a case of twisted nose.

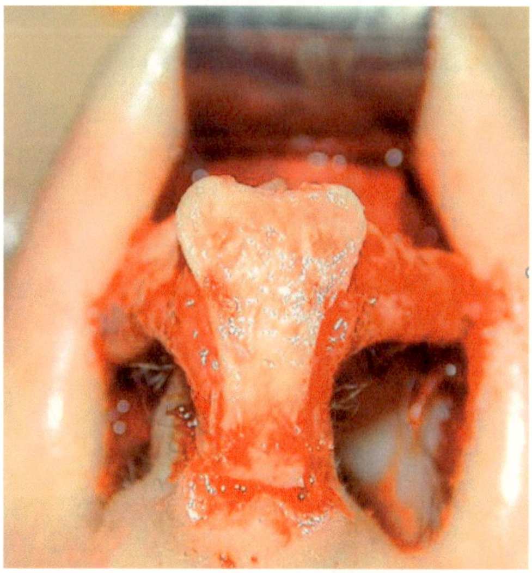

Figure 7.
Close-up view of shield graft augmentation tip plasty.

their sinus symptoms and were adequately satisfied with their nasal appearance. No revision rhinoplasty or ESS was performed on this group at the time of reporting.

There were no major complications noted in this study. There were minor complications reported which were mainly delayed wound healing [2], minor irregularities of the nasal dorsal skin lining [2], alar asymmetry [2], and pinching of the nose [1]. None of the patients were interested in further surgical intervention at that moment in time.

4. Discussion

In the population, there are patients with cosmetic nasal concerns who will also have functional problems (nasal obstruction and/or sinus problems) which should be fully evaluated. Moreover, patients with functional nasal problems would like a cosmetic nasal improvement (**Figures 8, 9**, and **10**). It is meaningful that patients who would benefit from rhinoplasty and ESS would wish to combine the two procedures which would save patients time, money, and inconvenience. Advances in powered sinus instrumentation have made combining rhinoplasty and ESS more attractive. In 1991, Sheman and Matarasso [15] first reported combining rhinoplasty and ESS, and since then various authors have reported a bigger series demonstrating the safety and efficacy of combining these two procedures [16–21].

Since the main complaint on presentation was chronic nasal obstruction (DNS with enlarged turbinates) with rhinosinusitis, all the patients had septal surgery with turbinate reduction. The CT scan of the paranasal sinuses performed on all the patients showed evidence of involvement of more than one paranasal sinus; the ESS was performed on more than one sinus. The most common sinuses involved were the ethmoid and the maxillary sinuses, with less incidence of involvement of sphenoid and frontal sinuses. Since all the patients presented with internal nasal valve problems, all the patients had spreader with shield graft performed.

Since all patients had caudal septal deviation with narrow nasal valve, spreader graft was performed on all patients. Only 24.5% of patients had mid-vault deformity which required osteotomy.

Powered instrumentation combining suction, irrigation, debridement, and cautery reduces surgical steps, operative time, and blood loss. IGS is a valuable

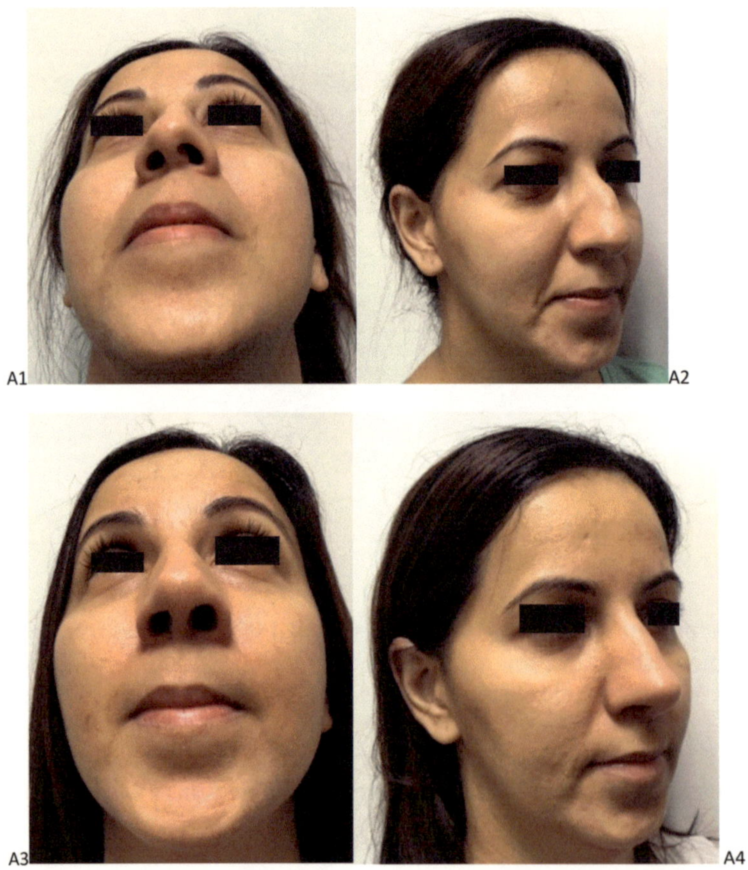

Figure 8.
Pre (A1 and A2) and postoperative (A3 and A4) pictures of patient no. 38 who presented with twisted nose, prominent nasal hump, and CRS.

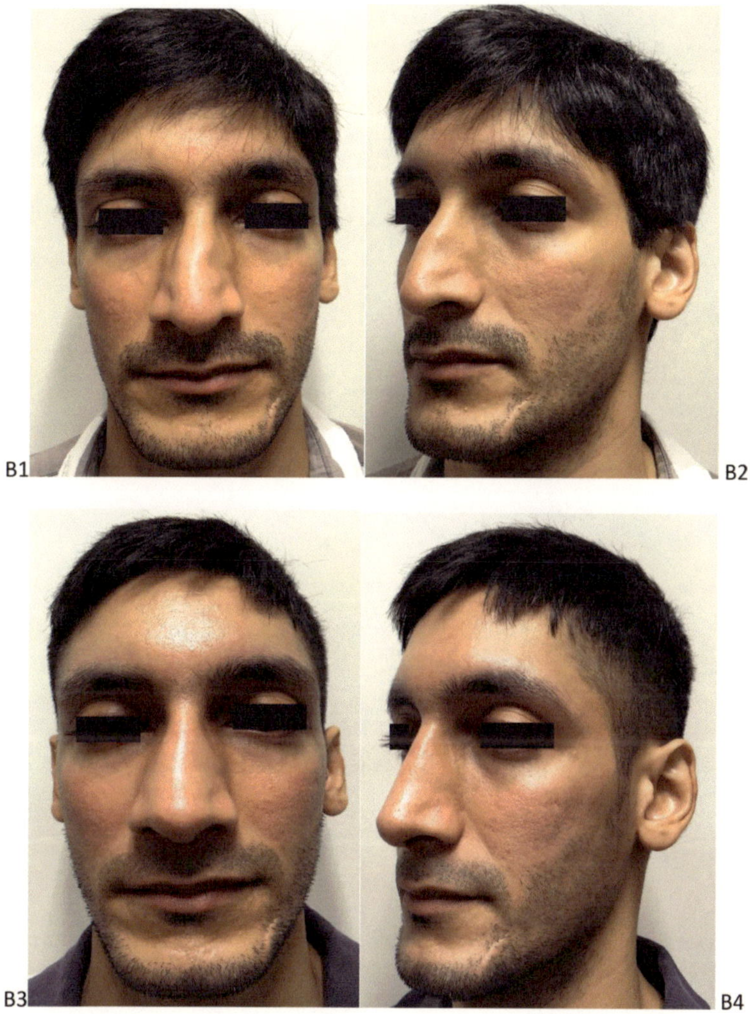

Figure 9.
Pre- (B1 and B2) and postoperative (B3 and B4) pictures of patient no. 13 who presented with crooked nose, pseudo-hump nasal hump, and CRS.

instrument used for anatomic confirmation especially in revision cases. Absorbable sinus packing has increased patient comfort. Advances in ESS instrumentation have made the procedure faster, safer, precise, and comfortable.

This addition of 53 cases of rhinoplasty with ESS to the literature by one surgeon technique illustrates the overall safety and efficacy of combining the two procedures. This study shows that the ESS using powered instrumentation is not too time-consuming, on average taking about 45 minutes in this study compared to 50 minutes in other reported cases [13]. Total blood loss for the combined procedure was about three times more (121 cc) in our study compared to blood loss in other studies (40 cc) [21] which could likely be due to the more extensive paranasal sinus mucosal disease involvement. The average operating time for the concurrent procedure was 186.20 minutes compared to 110 minutes in other reports [22] which could likely be due to time-consuming remodeling utilizing autografts. All the patients had some type of cartilage grafting with no evidence of infection, extrusion, malposition, or resorption since autologous grafts were used in all 53 patients. Minor complications like erythematous columellar incisions were treated aggressively with a course of oral antibiotics.

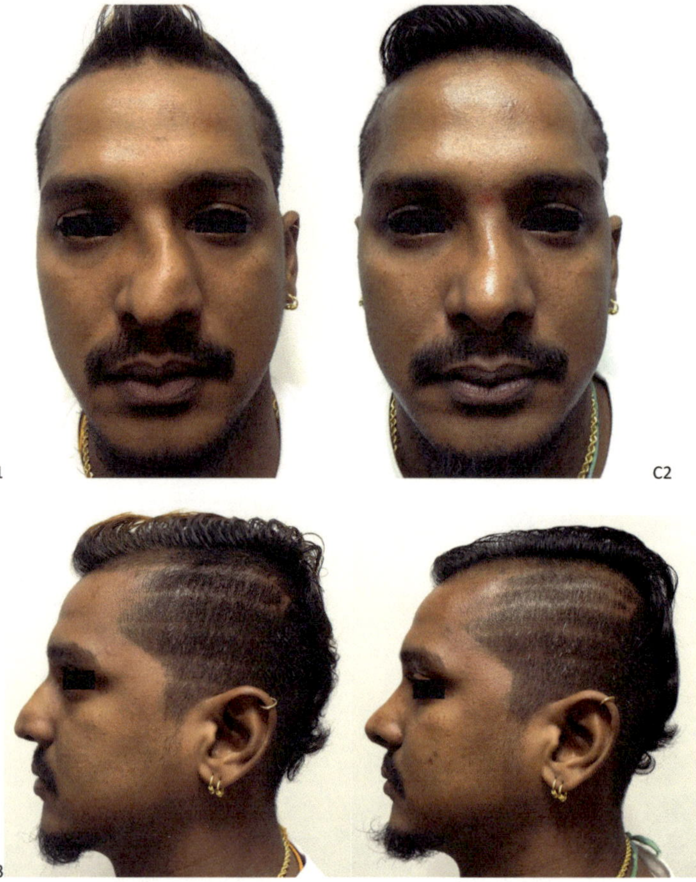

C1 C2 C3 C4

Figure 10.
Pre- (C1 and C2) and postoperative (C3 and C4) pictures of patient no. 26 who presented with twisted nose, pseudo-nasal hump, and CRS post-trauma.

A review of 268 rhinoplasties between 1997 and 2001 demonstrated 11 cases with concurrent surgery, and there were no complications noted in this study [17]. Furthermore, the authors mention a case report of a 22-year-old patient who underwent a septorhinoplasty and ESS on an outpatient basis at another institution and developed edema over the nose, cheek, glabella, and forehead regions with fever. A CT scan of paranasal sinuses showed evidence of opacification of the frontal sinuses with dehiscence of nasal bones which responded to intravenous medication and frontal trephination. Herzon in 1971 reported a 12% incidence of bacteremia in patients undergoing nasal septal surgery requiring nasal packing [23]. In 1978, Todd et al. reported the first case of toxic shock syndrome (TSS) [24].Four years later the first case of TSS after septorhinoplasty was reported [25].

Most authors agree that performing the sinus surgery first allows the surgeon to determine if there is ongoing rhinosinusitis. Millman B who performs combination rhinoplasty with ESS recommends not proceeding with rhinoplasty if there are signs of infection [17].

There have been only 4 reported cases of MRSA associated postoperative complications following septorhinoplasty reported in the literature across all specialities [26]. Patients who are susceptible to MRSA infections may also be at higher risk for nasal colonization, and this includes elderly patients, patients recently hospitalized or treated in a rehabilitation center, and health-care workers. Few cases of MRSA infection following septorhinoplasty have been reported in the literature. Elimination of nasal colonization is a major step in preventing these infections, and preoperative systemic antibiotic use should be considered, especially in revision cases [27].

Most of the sinus symptoms resolved postoperatively with 47 (88.6%) of 53 patients describing their improvement as significant. Fifty (94.3%) of 53 patients stated that they would recommend the concurrent procedure.

5. Conclusion

The author has reasonably good results combining rhinoplasty and ESS, and the benefits of these advances are illustrated by a review of the literature with good results (functional and cosmetic) and minimal complications. Extracorporeal approach was performed on all patients with gross high septal deviation. All the patients had some type of cartilage grafting with no evidence of infection, extrusion, malposition, or resorption since all the patients had autologous grafts inserted. Minor complications like erythematous columellar incisions were treated aggressively with a course of oral antibiotics. Advances in rhinoplasty and sinus surgery technique and equipment have made this one surgeon combined procedure safe and cost-effective with good results in selected patients.

Author details

Balwant Singh Gendeh
Pantai Hospital Kuala Lumpur, Kuala Lumpur, Malaysia

*Address all correspondence to: bsgendeh@gmail.com

References

[1] Murakami C. Nasal valve collapse. Ear, Nose, & Throat Journal. 2004;**83**:163-164

[2] Beekhuis GJ. Nasal obstruction after rhinoplasty: Etiology and techniques for correction. The Laryngoscope. 1976;**86**:540-548

[3] Scadding GK, Durham SR, Mirakian R, et al. BSACI guidelines for the management of rhinosinusitis and nasal polyposis. Clinical and Experimental Allergy. 2008;**38**(2):260-275

[4] Sheen JH. Spreader graft: A method of reconstructing the roof of the middle nasal vault following rhinoplasty. Plastic and Reconstructive Surgery. 1984;**73**(2):230-239

[5] Byrd HS, Andochick S, Copit S, et al. Septal extension grafts: A method of controlling tip projection shape. Plastic and Reconstructive Surgery. 1997;**100**:999-1010

[6] Whitaker EG, Johnson CM Jr. The evolution of open structure rhinoplasty. Archives of Facial Plastic Surgery. 2003;**5**:291-300. DOI: 10.1001/archfaci.5.4.291

[7] Toriumi DM. New concepts in nasal tip contouring. Archives of Facial Plastic Surgery. 2006;**8**:156-185. DOI: 10.1001/archfaci.8.3.156

[8] Clark JM, Cook TA. The "butterfly" graft in functional secondary rhinoplasty. Laryngoscope. 2002;**112**:1917-1925

[9] Lee DS, Glasgold AI. Correction of nasal valve stenosis with lateral suture suspension. Archives of Facial Plastic Surgery. 2001;**3**:237-240

[10] Schlosser RJ, Park SS. Surgery of the dysfunctional nasal valve: Cadaveric analysis and clinical outcomes. Archives of Facial Plastic Surgery. 1999;**1**:105-110

[11] Marchica P, Bassetto F, Vindigni V, Galici R, Dispenza F, Gallina S, et al. Endoscopic sinus surgery associated with rhinoseptoplasty: A case-control study. Plastic and Reconstructive Surgery Global Open. 2018;**10**:1-5

[12] Terrel JE. Primary sinus surgery. In: Cummings CW, Friedrickson JM, Harker LA, et al, editors. Otolaryngology Head Neck Surgery. Vol. 2. St Louis: Mosby; 1998. pp. 1160-1162

[13] Levine HL, May M, Schaitkin B, Mester SJ. Results of surgery. In: Levine H, May M, editors. Endoscopic Sinus Surgery. New York: Thieme Medical Publishes Inc; 1993. pp. 176-192

[14] Rizk SS, Edelstein DR, Matarasso A. Concurrent functional endoscopic sinus surgery and rhinoplasty. Annals of Plastic Surgery. 1997;**38**:323-329

[15] Sheman LJ, Matarasso A. Combined endoscopic sinus surgery and aesthetic rhinoplasty: A pilot study. American Journal of Rhinology. 1991;**5**:131-136

[16] Toffel PH. Simultaneous secure endoscopic sinus surgery and rhinoplasty. Ear, Nose and Throat Journal. 1994;**73**(8):554-573

[17] Milman B, Smith R. The potential pitfalls of concurrent rhinoplasty and endoscopic sinus surgery. Laryngoscope. 2002;**112**(71):1193-1196

[18] Mazzola RF, Felisati G. Rhinoplasty and endoscopic surgery for functional and inflammatory nasal/sinus disorders. Plastic and Reconstructive Surgery. 2005;**115**(3):705-710

[19] Lee JH, Sherris DA, Moore EJ. Combined open septorhinoplasty and

functional endoscopic sinus surgery. Otolaryngology. 2005;**133**(3):436-440

[20] Inanli S, Sari M, Yazici MZ. The results of concurrent functional endoscopic sinus surgery and rhinoplasty. The Journal of Craniofacial Surgery. 2008;**19**(3):701-704

[21] Marcus B, Patel Z, Busquets J, Hwang PH, Cook TA. The utility of concurrent rhinoplasty and sinus surgery: A 2-team approach. Archives of Facial Plastic Surgery. 2006;**8**(4):260-262

[22] Murrell GL. Rhinoplasty and functional endoscopic sinus surgery. Plastic Surgery International. 2011;**10**: 1-6. DOI: 10.155/2011/473481

[23] Herzon FS. Bacteremia and local infections with nasal packing. Archives of Otolaryngology. 1971;**94**:31-32

[24] Todd J, Fishaut M, Kapral F, Welch T. Toxic shock syndrome associated with phase group! *Staphylococcus*. Lancet. 1979;**1**:1116-1118

[25] Thomas SW, Baird IM, Frazier RD. Toxic shock syndrome following submucous resection and rhinoplasty. JAMA. 1982;**247**:2402-2403

[26] Lohr GD, Hollabaugh B, Waters P, Tiwana PS. Methicillin-resistant *Staphylococcus aureus* and antibiotic use in septorhinoplasty: Case report and review of literature. Journal of Oral Medicine, Oral Surgery, Oral Pathology and Oral Radiology. 2017;**123**(6):e 177-e 188

[27] Angelos PC, Wang TD. Methicillin-resistant *Staphylococcus aureus* infection in septorhinoplasty. Laryngoscope. 2010;**120**(7):1309-1311